D0122765

A WORLD BEYOND HEALING

Also by Nicholas Wade

THE ULTIMATE EXPERIMENT
THE NOBEL DUEL
BETRAYERS OF THE TRUTH

A WORLD BEYOND HEALING

The Prologue and Aftermath of Nuclear War

NICHOLAS WADE

W·W·NORTON & COMPANY

New York   London

First Edition

The text of this book is composed in Bodoni Book,
with display type set in Fenice Regular.
Composition and manufacturing by The Haddon Craftsmen, Inc.
Book design by Jacques Chazaud.

Library of Congress Cataloging-in-Publication Data
Wade, Nicholas.
A world beyond healing.
Includes index.
1. Nuclear warfare.   I.Title.
U263.W33   1987   355'.0217   86–21663

ISBN 0-393-02335-4

W. W. Norton & Company, Inc., 500 Fifth Avenue, New York, N. Y. 10110
W. W. Norton & Company Ltd., 37 Great Russell Street, London, WC1B 3NU

1 2 3 4 5 6 7 8 9 0

Contents

Preface

Many people believe that rational leaders will never let a nuclear war begin but that, should war happen, everyone will die. Neither belief is well founded.

New safety devices and procedures have eased the once substantial danger that a nuclear war might be triggered by a false warning of attack or the unintended launch of a nuclear weapon. Nor, from the clear blue sky, is one side at all likely to launch a surprise attack on the other; nuclear weapons are frightening enough to deter any such gamble. But there remain other paths to nuclear war that are not yet well enough guarded.

Perhaps the most dangerous is war by preemptive attack. In time of international crisis, one side might fear, correctly or not, that the other was about to launch a nuclear attack, and might decide it would be better to strike first than to hold its fire and hope to retaliate after riding out an attack. Thus crisis could ignite a nuclear war that neither side had intended. Millions would die in the exchange. But after the last missile had been fired, many millions of people in the belligerent states would still be alive.

How many of the survivors would also perish in the months and years ahead? What kind of world would the survivors face?

How long would economic reconstruction take? Governments that threaten—and are threatened by—nuclear retaliation cannot be indifferent to the consequences if deterrence should fail. Yet, in a strangely consistent pattern, governments have been reluctant to ascertain the full destructive powers of the awesome weapons they wield.

The issue is clouded by contention as well as ignorance. Defense analysts who fret that the public may turn against nuclear weapons and demand unilateral disarmament tend to minimize their effects, sometimes to bizarre extremes. A senior Defense Department official, T. K. Jones, preached in 1981 that the United States could fully recover from an all-out nuclear exchange in four years or less, provided that Americans built homemade dirt shelters against radiation. "If there are enough shovels to go around, everybody's going to make it," he said. At the other extreme are those who exaggerate the effects of nuclear war—difficult though that is to do—in order to buttress the case for particular disarmament proposals. Worldwide famine, raging epidemics, collective psychoses, even the spread of AIDS, are among the wilder speculations that some scientists have confidently announced for the aftermath of nuclear war.

As Edward Zuckerman notes in *The Day after World War III,* "Most arguments about the effects of nuclear war thus tend to be political arguments in the guise of scientific arguments. . . . Those preaching the dangers of ozone depletion are attempting to win converts not only to their theories of exo-atmospheric chemistry but also to their views about the best way to manage the arms race and arms control negotiations. Those who minimize the effects of nuclear war tend to have different views."

The purpose of this book is to present a concise and impartial account of nuclear war—how a nuclear war might start; what nuclear weapons do to people, cities, and the natural environment; and what the chances are of economic and ecological recovery in the aftermath of a nuclear exchange. The book reviews recent thinking about the causes and effects of nuclear war. It seeks to remedy the neglect of those awkward factors that often seem to find little place in the strategists' abstract discussions of nuclear war. These include the psychology of leaders during crisis, the vulnerability of the communications through which national leaders command and control their strategic nuclear forces, the nuclear electromagnetic pulse and its ability to derange electrical equipment over vast areas, the superfires that may be ignited by the thermal pulse of nuclear weapons in stricken cities, the climatic changes induced by the smoke of a nuclear exchange, and the impact of such effects on people and their surroundings. In particular, I have tried to assess the evidence skeptically, to stress uncertainties in present scientific knowledge where they exist, and to avoid both understatement and exaggeration.

In the last world war, some 50 million people perished. For more than four decades so far, the policy of nuclear deterrence has successfully prevented another such a war. Yet the policy entails a fearful risk—of nuclear catastrophe should deterrence fail. The government laboratories and scientists that design nuclear weapons have not always taken the lead in exploring their adverse effects.

The phenomenon of radioactive fallout was not seriously studied until after 1954, when a test explosion unexpectedly contaminated 7,000 square miles of the Marshall Islands area of the Pacific with lethal amounts of radioactivity. The weapons establishments of the world's nuclear powers were again apparently taken by surprise over the threat that nuclear weapons pose to the earth's ozone layer, the invisible atmospheric shield that protects animals and plants from ultraviolet light. Scientists studying a proposed supersonic passenger plane noted in 1973 that the ozone layer could be depleted by the exhaust gases known as nitrogen oxides. Only then was it remembered that nuclear weapons produce nitrogen oxides in profusion from the air they explode in and that these gases can ascend to the ozone layer.

Another overlooked nuclear side effect, the phenomenon known as nuclear winter, was perhaps the most obvious of all. It is no secret that Hiroshima and Nagasaki burned. Burning cities create soot, and soot absorbs light. If enough smoke from incinerated cities were to reach high enough in the atmosphere, it might linger for months, shrouding the earth in a black pall. The likely extent of such a veil is still a matter of keen scientific debate, but an evident possibility is that sunlight would be blotted out, land and crops throughout the Northern Hemisphere chilled, and whole harvests destroyed.

The void of knowledge left by government scientists has slowly been filled in and the information disseminated to a wider public, often by scientists with no professional interest in nuclear warfare. A well-researched but apocalyptic series of *New Yorker* articles by Jonathan Schell in 1981, later published as *The Fate of the Earth*, introduced many readers to the panoply of different physical catastrophes that are set in train by a nuclear explosion. The hypothesis of the nuclear winter effect, first suggested in 1983 and popularized in *The Cold and the Dark*, by Carl Sagan and Paul Ehrlich, prompted a resurgence of interest among civilian scientists in the climatic effects of nuclear war. A wide-ranging review of all aspects of nuclear war, both biological and physical, was issued in 1985 by the SCOPE committee of the International Council of Scientific Unions. A review conference of similar breadth was held in September 1985 by the Institute of Medicine in Washington, D.C.*

As the new reappraisals make evident, the effects of nuclear

---

*At the suggestion of the publisher, this book was to have presented a version for the general reader of the Institute of Medicine's conference. In the course of preparation, however, it evolved into an independent account, drawing on many sources besides the institute's conference.

weapons may be even more far reaching than hitherto supposed. Some may take that as an argument for improving deterrence and civil defense measures or constructing a defense against nuclear missiles; others, as an urgent reason for more arms control and fewer new strategic weapons.

The effects of nuclear weapons do not make for pleasant reading. But the paradox of why we need weapons too terrible ever to be used deserves understanding. Not until that understanding is acquired will the task of abolishing them be likely to succeed.

A WORLD BEYOND HEALING

1

Under the Shadow

Today Hiroshima and Nagasaki are thriving modern cities. Monuments apart, there are no signs of the events of August 1945. Visitors find it hard to connect such a past with the flourishing scene before their eyes. The physical scars of war, even nuclear scars, have completely healed.

But the pall from the nuclear weapons that fell on Hiroshima and Nagasaki has never dissipated. The world's two superpowers conduct their relations under its immanent shadow. The threat of nuclear retaliation is the cornerstone of each superpower's defense against the other. The United States and the Soviet Union have worked continually to improve their strategic forces and make the threat of nuclear war ever more credible. Lesser countries seek to wield the same symbols of power. Britain, France, and China have advanced weapons and means of delivery; half a dozen other nations stand poised to step across the threshold to nuclear weaponry.

Deterrence has succeeded—so far. The structure of deterrence is in some ways reassuring. The superpowers have developed rules for conducting their diplomatic confrontations. In times of crisis, each avoids taking irrevocable positions. All

confrontations in the last 40 years have been successfully concluded without hostilities between American and Soviet forces.
Arms control negotiations stretching over many years have given
each side an intimate glimpse into the nature of the other's
strategic forces and thinking. The treaties that result may have
moderated the accumulation of nuclear weaponry only slightly,
but the process of negotiation is in itself a valuable bridge
between otherwise suspicious and implacable adversaries.

But in other ways the stability of deterrence is eroding. Technical progress had created missiles of greater accuracy and ver-
satility. Soviet submarines in the Atlantic, American missiles in
Europe, can each devastate the other's capital or command centers within a few minutes of being launched. As a first strike
attack seems capable of putting increasingly more of a nation's
nuclear forces and command structure at risk, the incentive to
attack first in crisis becomes more compelling.

Making Decisions under Stress

In confrontations between nuclear-armed adversaries, the decisions taken by political leaders are of the utmost importance:
mistakes are liable to be irretrievable. The machinery of government and of the complex military organizations that control
nuclear forces is particularly difficult for a single leader or executive group to keep under control.

The speed and volume of modern telecommunications presents decision makers with an extraordinary burden of information. In a fast-developing crisis, the burden may become intolerable to some individuals and may force others into errors of
judgment.

If a nuclear attack should be detected, the time for decisions
would be so short as to allow little deviation from prearranged
contingency plans. Intercontinental land-based missiles may be
detected by satellites a minute or so after launch, and their flight
time is 25 to 30 minutes. The time for decision making is likely

to be even less, since an adversary would doubtless precede such an attack with the launching of missiles from nearby submarines. Soviet submarine missiles could create havoc with American communications as little as four minutes after launch, and might detonate over land-based targets within 10 minutes.

Decision making in a nuclear war would be difficult enough even if the President had full access to information and if the command and control system were left intact. But a Soviet attack is likely to be aimed at destroying the sensors and communications system on which the President would hope to rely in making decisions. Even if the President escaped to the National Emergency Airborne Command Post, a plane equipped with the communications to control American nuclear forces, the information available to him would become increasingly partial and confused. The President and his advisers would have to confer with the commander of the Strategic Air Command and other officers, seek confirmation of the attack, and authorize an appropriate response.

A rational and considered decision under the conditions of nuclear attack seems difficult at best. According to Richard K. Betts, "Too many things would have to happen within twenty-five minutes or less: tactical warning would have to be processed through the chain of command; the President would have to hear it, believe it, and authorize firing; the authorization would have to be transmitted back and confirmed to missile crews, who would have to believe it and then turn their keys. On paper, this can all be accomplished within the time available; in the heat of crisis, with terrified people facing apocalypse, such a smooth-flowing sequence is scarcely conceivable. . . . In one or more links of the chain of command, people are likely to disbelieve, panic, or wait and demand reconfirmation."[1]

Even before the missiles started to fly, a major political confrontation between the United States and the Soviet Union would severely tax, maybe overwhelm, the managerial capacities of decision makers, no matter how psychologically stable or politically skilled. The low level military actions and interactions of the nuclear command organizations on each side could not be predicted or controlled in all their important details. A redirection of photoreconnaissance satellites in response to a crisis would be detected by one side and prompt a response, which would be detected by the other, and so forth in an escalating spiral. These low-level behaviors of military organizations are far too extensive and elaborate for anyone in central authority to control in detail. Mutual interactions might occur so fast that they would outpace and tend to dominate the normal diplomatic channels used to negotiate a constructive resolution. For example, if Soviet nuclear submarines started to leave port, American reconnaissance satellites would detect the movement and American military commanders would insist on making the necessary countermoves.

The tension between the diplomatic goal of negotiation and the military objective of striking first would inevitably produce major differences in judgment between the civilian and political leadership on both sides, making it very difficult for rapid and consistent lines of action to be established.[2]

Given their shared fear of nuclear war, American and Soviet leaders have strong motives to conclude diplomatic crises before they risk losing control of events and to abide by the general principles and operational requirements of crisis management. Most individuals who reach high-level policy-making positions have probably learned to cope with decisional stress and are emotionally stable. The severe mental illness that afflicted Secretary of Defense James Forrestal is an exception. But the cumulative emotional strain and physical fatigue imposed by a prolonged crisis can severely drain participants.

Historical accounts of American policy-making during the Cuban missile crisis have long hinted at the effects of stress on the decision-making group. A member of the group, Theodore Sorensen, wrote cryptically that he had seen at first hand, during the long days and nights of the crisis, "how brutally physical and mental fatigue can numb the good sense as well as the senses of normally articulate men." Robert Kennedy made a similar observation in his memoir of the episode: "That kind of crisis-induced pressure does strange things to a human being, even to brilliant, self-confident, mature, experienced men. For some it brings out characteristics and strengths that perhaps even they never knew they had, and for others the pressure is too over-whelming." Recently a former high official in the Kennedy Administration told the political scientist Alexander George that two important members of the President's advisory group had been unable to cope with the stress. They became quite passive and were unable to fulfill their responsibilities. Their condition become so evident that others took over their duties. Yet the performance of the policy-making group as a whole during the missile crisis is generally regarded as having been of high order.[3]

Inability to cope with the stress of political crises is not so rare. Stalin evidently suffered a temporary depression after the Nazi invasion of the Soviet Union in 1941. In the wake of Britain's disastrous invasion of Suez in Egypt in 1956, Prime Minister Anthony Eden suffered a near physical and emotional collapse. In the prolonged crisis preceding Israel's attack on Egypt and Syria in 1967, Army Chief of Staff Yitzhak Rabin was temporarily relieved of his duties because of the effects of stress and nicotine poisoning. Prime Minister Jawaharlal Nehru was mentally and physically incapacitated in the aftermath of India's defeat by China in 1962, as was Gamal Abdel Nasser after Egypt's defeat in 1967.

The stress of crisis may impair the performance of groups as well as of individuals. It is a familiar pattern for groups under pressure to discourage and shut out members who raise disturbing questions that may undermine the group's confidence in its proposed solutions. President Johnson's policy-making group on the Vietnam War took on some of the characteristics of a body seeking to protect itself from critical views.[4]

The policy of nuclear deterrence has secured a peace between the superpowers that probably could not have been maintained for so long by any other means. Yet the peace has been bought by incurring a risk that grows steadily less favorable. Not only does the chance of miscalculation increase with each year that passes, but the technology-driven evolution of nuclear weapons systems imposes increasingly difficult choices on decision makers. Before the advent of the intercontinental ballistic missile, the bombers that carried each side's nuclear weapons could in principle be launched in a crisis and later recalled. Now the time available for critical decisions has shrunk from hours to minutes. The chances for errors of judgment are far greater, and the consequences, as explored in the following chapters, are extraordinarily severe.

2

The Fragilities of Command and Control

The United States and the Soviet Union have both created large and complex organizations to manage their nuclear forces. The behavior of these organizations is of critical importance in both peace and war: in peace to resist false alarms and prevent the accidental launch of weapons, in war to execute intended commands and maintain leaders' control over their forces.

For 40 years peacetime control of nuclear weapons has been safely exercised. That gives some ground for confidence, little for complacency. As procedures and machinery become more complex, false alerts can occur in new and more insidious ways. A more serious uncertainty is the behavior of governments in crises. An evident risk is that an unintended war might be set off by an escalating series of interactions between the two superpowers. Compounding that risk is the incentive that each side would have for striking first, should war come to seem inevitable. The policy of nuclear deterrence, in other words, is vulnerable to catastrophic failure.

The Nuclear Force Structure

The United States and the Soviet Union each possess about 10,000 nuclear warheads in their strategic arsenals, deliverable by bombers and by missiles launched from land-based silos and from submarines. The Soviet Union's strategic force is heavily concentrated in its land-based missiles, many of which are deployed with multiple warheads. These 1,398 missiles carry 6,-420 warheads. The Soviet Union possesses 946 submarine-launched missiles, carrying 2,122 warheads, and 303 strategic bombers, capable of delivering 1,052 warheads.

The United States has chosen to spread its nuclear weapons more evenly among the three arms, or triad, of its strategic force. Its 1,030 land-based missiles carry 2,130 warheads. The 592 submarine-launched missiles can deliver 5,344 warheads. And 297 American bombers carry bombs or air-launched cruise missiles with a total of 3,296 warheads.[1]

Soviet warheads have larger yields, ranging from 0.2 megatons (200 kilotons) up to a massive 24 megatons. American missiles, being more accurate, do not need such large explosive power to destroy their targets. Apart from the 9-megaton warheads of the venerable Titan missiles, now being retired, almost all American warheads are of 1 megaton or less. Both superpowers have reduced the yields of their warheads as the accuracy of delivery vehicles has increased.[2]

The plethora of weapons and warheads stems from the different advantages and purposes of each. Land-based missiles have greater accuracy than sea-launched missiles and in a crisis can reach their targets (often other land-based missiles) more quickly than can bombers. But land-based missiles, even when protected in hardened silos, are thought to be vulnerable to attack. Each side also relies on submarine-based missiles. Satellites can monitor submarines in port, and submarines can be detected as they pass certain fixed sonar arrays. But there is no general method for detecting submarines at sea, and no immediate likelihood of any technical advance that would make the oceans transparent. Unless tracked from port or otherwise located, missile-carrying submarines are undetectable when at sea and hence invulnerable.

Submarine-launched missiles are less accurate than land-based missiles and at present lack the ability to destroy hardened missile silos. The D5 missile due to be installed on American Trident submarines in the late 1980s will be the first sea-based weapon to have an accuracy comparable to that of land-based missiles.

Bombers are soft targets, very vulnerable to attack. They are slow to deliver their weapons and may suffer attrition from the opponent's air defenses. Nonetheless, they possess the considerable advantage of being able to be recalled after launch. They also provide a proven method of delivery, whereas modern strategic missiles, although exhaustively tested over practice ranges, have never been used in warfare.

This powerful triad of nuclear forces is under the control of an elaborate command structure. The nuclear command structure receives considerably less attention than do the weapons it wields, yet its behavior is critical to the initiation and outcome of any nuclear conflict. The nuclear command structure integrates many different elements, from satellites that give warning of Soviet missiles leaving their silos to airborne command posts that would relay orders to retaliate.

At the organizational center of the structure is the President and the National Military Command Center, located in the Pentagon, in Washington. Since Washington might be an early target of Soviet attack, there exists an Alternate National Military Command Center, at Fort Ritchie, Maryland. There is also an airborne command post for the President, an EC-135 aircraft stationed at Andrews Air Force Base, in Washington. The plane, able to take off at 15 minutes' warning, is known as the National Emergency Airborne Command Post. Another major strategic center is the North American Aerospace Defense Command, situated within Cheyenne Mountain, Colorado.

An elaborate worldwide system of technical devices feeds information into these command centers, and a complex communications system carries instructions from the centers to the nuclear weapons under their control. The input to the system comes from radars, early warning satellites, and intelligence agencies like the National Security Agency, which specializes in eavesdropping on Soviet communications and signals traffic. The radars include the Perimeter Acquisition Radar Control System, north of Grand Forks, North Dakota, which can track Soviet missiles on trajectories over the North Pole and accurately predict their targets. The PAVE PAWS radars on the Atlantic and Pacific coasts are designed to give warning of attacks by missiles launched from submarines.

Satellites in orbit over Soviet missile fields are equipped to detect the heat of the rocket boosters as they leave their silos. The 30 minutes or so of warning time provided by these satellites, and the 10 or so minutes that might be given by the radars, is known as tactical warning. This is different from strategic warning, which would give one or two days' warning of an attack. Strategic warning comes from detection of the "alerting fingerprint"—the flurry of communications traffic generated when the opponent puts his nuclear forces on alert. It is important to note that strategic warning constitutes a channel through which the nuclear command structures of the two sides interact with one another. When one side puts its forces on alert, or switches its planes and ships from general intelligence to tactical intelligence, the other side will detect the change and may make a corresponding disposition. This creates the danger of an escalating series of interactive alerts.

The output from the nuclear command structures is almost as complex as the input. The executive organizations that control the nuclear forces are the Strategic Air Command, in charge of bombers and land-based missiles, and the Navy's Atlantic and

Pacific Commands, CINCLANT and CINCPAC, which control the nuclear missile carrying submarine fleets. Numerous communication links, from hardened ground lines to radio stations and satellites, tie the elements of the command structure together. Almost all are vulnerable to nuclear attack, in particular to an esoteric effect of nuclear weapons known as the electromagnetic pulse.

The fallback communications link in event of attack is a fleet of airborne command posts, known as the Post Attack Command Control System, or PACCS. The PACCS aircraft are intended to relay radio communications between one another and to bombers and missile command posts. If the President or surviving political authority were aboard the National Emergency Airborne Command Post, the PACCS aircraft would provide radio communications linking him with Looking Glass, the alternative airborne command post for the Strategic Air Command, and with the airborne command posts for the Navy's CINCLANT and CINCPAC. A second fleet of aircraft, known as TACAMO, provide communications with submarines on alert status.[3]

The Accidental Path to Nuclear War

In January 1961 a B-52 bomber carrying two high yield nuclear weapons crashed south of Goldsboro, North Carolina. In one bomb the accident detonated the conventional explosive charge that drives the nuclear material into a critical mass, but safety devices prevented a nuclear explosion. In the other bomb all the safety interlocks were triggered but one. Had the last interlock been thrown, the nuclear weapon would have detonated.[4]

Aside from the damage to a country's own territory, an accidental nuclear explosion could induce a government to believe it was under attack. An even more serious accident would be the inadvertent or unauthorized launch of a nuclear weapon. How safe are nuclear weapons?

American nuclear weapons are embedded in a carefully designed complex of safety systems intended to forestall every conceivable misadventure that might lead to unintended detonation. These include fire, flood, explosion, electromagnetic effects, terrorists, enemy capture, psychopathic insiders, and even a hard-pressed military crew trying to cut corners on an authorized launch.[5]

A nuclear weapon is detonated by arranging for a spherical outer shell of conventional high explosive to be ignited at all points simultaneously. The explosion compresses the nuclear material within the sphere so that it attains criticality. Nuclear weapons are now designed with "one-point safety." If the conventional explosive is ignited at one point, as by fire or by being dropped, the nuclear material will not go critical.

The electrical system that orders the detonation of the weapon is kept separate from the system with the nuclear materials, and both are packaged in an "exclusion" region designed to protect them from fire, shock, chemicals, high current, and the electromagnetic effects of nuclear blasts. The exclusion region may fail against these threats, but before it does, the deliberately weak link between the detonation system and the nuclear system is designed to fail first.

Nuclear weapons are equipped with an environmental sensing device (ESD) that monitors the environments that the warhead is expected to traverse between launch and detonation. The ESD in a nuclear bomb will check for the zero gravity of free-fall, then for the arresting motion of a parachute. On missile warheads the ESD may look for the vacuum of space or the deceleration of reentry. Detonation is prevented if the ESD fails to detect the expected conditions.

Nuclear devices are usually enclosed in an internally powered membrane with sensors to detect unauthorized attempts at penetration. Depending on the nature of the attempt, the warhead will be automatically disabled or destroyed.

All warheads except those on Navy ships carry permissive action links (PALs), which are designed to make possession and control of the weapon two quite separate matters. Whoever may possess the weapon, it can be detonated only if a code is received from appropriate authorities and used to unlock an electronic combination lock in the warhead's circuitry. Terrorists, errant insiders, or hostile military forces who might capture a warhead will be incapable of detonating it without the code that unlocks the PAL.

The need for PALs on sea-borne warheads is less severe, since ships and submarines are unlikely to be captured except in circumstances that would give the crew time to disable or destroy them. The difficulty of communicating with ships and submarines is another reason for not installing PALs, because the enabling codes might not get through when needed. Instead of PALs, the Navy relies on launch check lists to prevent unauthorized launch. Any message to launch nuclear weapons must be announced to the entire crew and verified by two teams of officers. Keys are then issued to other officers responsible for launch, who must turn their keys in a prescribed sequence.

Another layer of safeguards lies in various personnel procedures. The "two-man" rule requires every sensitive action with nuclear weapons to be undertaken by two people. Around every nuclear weapon are "no-lone zones," where no one is allowed to go unaccompanied. People with access to nuclear weapons are checked for drug abuse and psychiatric problems through a Personnel Reliability Program. Finally, the containers used to store and transport nuclear weapons are equipped with sensors that may respond to unauthorized penetrations by isolating the weapons and immobilizing the entrants.

These devices and procedures, the fruit of much thought and experience, are a considerable achievement. They have resulted, notes Donald Cotter, in "a flawless record of nuclear safety."[6]

False Alerts

False alerts are another serious but, so far, manageable threat to nuclear stability in peacetime. False alerts are in fact recognized as being so serious that the nuclear command organizations are primed to respond to alerts with great caution.

In the 1950s a flock of Canadian geese was reportedly misinterpreted by the DEW Line early warning radar network as an attack by Soviet bombers. In 1979, a serious false alert occurred at the North American Aerospace Defense Command (NORAD), inside Cheyenne Mountain in Colorado. An erroneous message transmitted because of an operator's error was sent to NORAD fighter bases. Several fighters were scrambled, and missile and submarine bases across the nation switched to a higher state of alert.

A similar false alert occurred a few months later through failure of a 46-cent computer chip in a NORAD computer. About a hundred B-52 bombers and the President's National Emergency Airborne Command Post were readied for takeoff, and the airborne command post of the U.S. commander in the Pacific actually took off.

These two false alerts led to further procedural and technical changes to reduce the risk. Many believe the dangers of false alerts are now well controlled. In peacetime, notes John Steinbruner, "the dominant objective of the managerial system is that of preventing any unauthorized use of even an individual weapon. Elaborate and so far very successful procedures have been worked out within all military systems to guarantee that negative control can be exercised under all situations normally encountered. We have lived for more than 20 years successfully under those arrangements."[7] A similar conclusion is reached by Paul Bracken of Yale University: "Against the discrete accident, malfunction, or operator error the total system is massively redundant. . . . I believe the likelihood of nuclear war by pure technical accident is much lower today than it was twenty years ago, precisely because of today's more complex warning and control system."[8]

Similar procedures for preventing an unauthorized launch are thought to be in effect in the Soviet Union. Soviet nuclear depots are under the command of the KGB, the internal police, and nuclear forces are tied to the political leadership in Moscow by two separate links, one military and one KGB. According to Stephen Meyer, there is some evidence that missile launch control centers are manned by a crew of four, two KGB and two military. This indicates a concern on the part of the Soviet leadership to maintain tight control over nuclear forces and to guard against unauthorized and accidental use. In addition, Soviet missiles are now equipped with electronic locks, as are American missiles.[9]

False Alerts in Crisis

In the 1960s the danger of stumbling into nuclear war by accident was probably quite considerable. The technical and procedural safeguards adopted by the Defense Department have substantially reduced this danger. These measures constitute what is known as negative control. In times of crisis, however, the priorities of the nuclear command structure change and the procedures of negative control are replaced with those of positive control. The need to ensure that weapons are not launched accidentally yields to the need to ensure that they will be launched if the President or his successor so commands.

No one knows how smoothly the transition from negative to positive control would be accomplished. Even if everything worked as planned, the danger of false alerts would become markedly higher as the procedures of positive control switched into place.

The Paths to Nuclear War

Analysts often recognize five ways in which nuclear war might start. Accidental war is one. Another is catalytic war, in which use of nuclear weapons by third parties, whether nations or terrorist groups, draws the superpowers into direct conflict. A third route is by escalation of conventional war. Should a conventional war start in Europe between the forces of NATO and the Warsaw pact, one side might resort to use of tactical nuclear weapons, the term given to short-range weapons used on the European battlefield. Use of tactical nuclear weapons runs a high chance of inducing a strategic nuclear war between the United States and the Soviet Union.

A fourth way to nuclear war is surprise attack: a bolt from the blue attack by one superpower with no precipitating crisis. Fifth is preemptive attack, a strike launched during an international confrontation because one side believes, rightly or wrongly, that the other is about to strike first. All paths to nuclear war are unlikely, but the least improbable is preemptive attack in crisis.

Accidental war, as discussed above, was once a serious likelihood but has now been brought under substantial control. Catalytic war will become more likely if more nations develop nuclear weapons but at present is a somewhat theoretical danger. A conventional war between the superpowers is so evidently likely to lead to nuclear war that both are well deterred; the purpose of nuclear deterrence is to prevent conventional as well as nuclear war. Surprise attack is unlikely for the same reason. However successfully a surprise attack were executed, the aggressor would suffer a devastating setback from even the most ragged retaliatory strike.

The conditions in which leaders might contemplate a preemptive strike are quite different, because then they have reason to believe they may be attacked anyway. The choice is whether to risk riding out a nuclear attack or to strike first. The nature of nuclear command structures offers important incentives for striking first.

The Incentives for Preemptive Attack

In an international crisis a superpower afraid that its adversary might attack would have two strong reasons to strike first. Both arise from the weakness of the superpowers' nuclear command structures. These elaborate organizations are so vulnerable that a leader who does not strike first may well fear losing the power to strike at all. Conversely, by striking first, he may hope to paralyze the adversary's power of retaliation. At the least, he may gamble that the adversary's counterblow will be measurably less savage than an unimpaired first strike.

The nuclear command structure is interwoven with overlapping communication links. How could it be so paralyzed as to prevent or even substantially impair the execution of the order to retaliate? Communications equipment is particularly vulnerable to the nuclear weapons effect known as the electromagnetic pulse. A nuclear weapon exploded high in the atmosphere can create strong currents and high voltages at ground level for many hundreds of miles in all directions. The pulse can damage any electrical and electronic equipment that has not been specially protected, including radio, radar, telephone, and telegraph systems and computers. Because the pulse is likely to disrupt many communications systems and land lines, airborne command posts would be the mainstay of the nuclear command structure in war, but both the airplanes themselves and the radio communications between them are vulnerable to disruption in a nuclear environment. The chances that the President or his successors could transmit precise orders—fire these weapons, withhold those until further orders, cancel that launch to allow negotiations—will be small if the means of commanding the nuclear forces is in chaos.

The command structure could in some experts' view be so

severely shattered by a first strike that the coherence of retaliation might be significantly degraded. There are no more than
400 primary and secondary targets in the American nuclear
command structure, and the Soviets could easily afford to assign
two warheads to each. Targets would include the 100 launch
control centers from which the land-based Minutemen missiles
would be fired, the 14 ground entry points of the airborne
command posts, the 30 Navy and Air Force fixed radio stations
for communicating with the planes, the emergency rocket-borne
communications system, and the 15 ground-based primary and
alternate command centers.[10]

In the knowledge that the Soviet Union has the capacity to
destroy all ground-based communications, the United States depends on airborne command posts to carry out its second strike
retaliation. These include the President's airplane, the National
Emergency Airborne Command Post, as well as those of the
commanders of the Pacific and Atlantic commands, and the Air
Force and Navy planes designed to issue radio commands to the
Minuteman missile fields, the strategic bomber force, and nuclear submarines.

Even if these airplanes escape destruction on the ground from
submarine-launched missiles fired with just a few minutes' warning time, only the two planes assigned to the National Emergency Airborne Command Post are hardened against the electromagnetic pulse; all others lack protection. The planned launch
of a new generation of hardened satellites could considerably
improve the survival of communications in the future.

The risk of a Soviet attack that could block American retaliation would be lower under crisis conditions, because the United
States would already have started the transition from negative
to positive control of its nuclear forces. Nevertheless, says Bruce
Blair, "Even the theoretical optimum performance of past and
present [command and control] networks has not been sufficient
to ensure positive control. Deficiencies in communications that
have plagued the airborne network have by themselves greatly

undermined U.S. capabilities for retaliation. A Soviet first strike on an alert U.S. command system could still isolate most forces and severely reduce the effectiveness of the rest. . . . At present, notwithstanding a strong inclination to administer punishment swiftly, the state of U.S. [command and control] casts fundamental doubt on the ability of the United States to respond at all to Soviet nuclear attack."[11]

The Soviet command and control system is thought to be somewhat better protected, but not by enough to make any significant difference. The vulnerability of the command systems of both sides has two consequences. First, their weakness invites attack; second, the military commanders of the country under attack or threat of attack would have fierce incentives to launch all weapons under their command while they still had the ability to do so. "Whatever the declared national security policy in peacetime," notes Steinbruner, "the incentive appears to impose on responsible military commanders in both the U.S. and the U.S.S.R. potentially overwhelming pressures for outright preemption under intense crisis circumstances when the prospect of an unavoidable war would be facing them."[12]

Anything less than an all-out response to attack is improbable, because the means of assessing the scale of an opponent's strike is likely to be damaged along with the command and control system. "These circumstances," writes Blair, "encourage comprehensive retaliation. A limited Soviet counterforce attack [aimed at American nuclear forces] would not be unambiguously limited, and it would trigger pre-planned operations that, in conjunction with extensive collateral damage to the command system, would create strong pressures for organizing retaliation around a single plan that release most of the . . . retaliatory forces."[13] This pressure for comprehensive retaliation conflicts with the current American doctrine of flexible response, which calls for retaliation no stronger than necessary to deter the aggressor from further escalation. The purpose of this important policy is that, if deterrence should fail, nuclear war should be concluded at the lowest possible level of violence.

Escalation to Preemption

Since the danger of inciting a preemptive attack by the adversary is so evident, both superpowers tend to behave with extreme caution during periods of international crisis. Despite the recognized need for caution, there is still the risk that unintended or unauthorized actions by one superpower will induce a response by the other, triggering an escalating series of interactive hostilities. The nuclear command structures are so complex that no individual can control every detail of their operation.

Nuclear command organizations in crisis adjust their managerial balance from negative to positive control. The changes are brought about by standardized routines and programmed rules, all carefully thought out in advance. Yet, despite the planning, the changes cannot be completely determined or centrally controlled.

The reason is that operational procedures are too complex, too widely dispersed, and too responsive to the immediate circumstances of particular commanders for central control to be feasible. Some behaviors are preplanned, others depend on commanders following military tradition to bridge gaps in their instructions—for example, by aggressively seeking out the enemy in periods of alert. The result may depart significantly from the political authority's wishes.

There have been only two political crises involving the alert of strategic nuclear forces in the postwar period, those involving Cuba in 1962 and the Middle East in 1973. Both were marked by significant failures of managerial direction.

In the Cuban crisis, extraordinary and largely effective measures were undertaken to coordinate the actions of the American government and ensure that no military moves were made without express authority from the Executive. Yet a reconnaissance plane made an unauthorized incursion into Soviet airspace. It was officially described as an accident and was clearly unintended, at least by top managers.

An even more serious departure was the aggressive antisubmarine warfare operations conducted by the Navy against the Soviet submarines in the North Atlantic. The operations followed the Navy's standing rules of engagement but were not made known to the President and his senior advisers who were trying to manage the crisis. The Navy's campaign "constituted extremely strong strategic coercion and violated the spirit of the Executive Committee policy. It is not unreasonable to suppose that American [antisubmarine warfare] activity in the North Atlantic was in fact the strongest message perceived in Moscow in the course of the crisis and, if that is true, then the efforts to bring American policy under central direction must be said to have failed."[14]

In the Middle East crisis of 1973, an alert of nuclear forces was ordered by the U.S. Executive for the sole purpose of sending a secret diplomatic signal to the Soviet Union. Those who ordered the alert knew little about what they were ordering: they believed they could keep it from becoming public. It became public very rapidly.

The unintended actions of a nuclear command structure in crisis are of particular concern because of the effect they have on that of the other side. The early warning systems of each carefully monitor and react to the actions of the other. Reconnaissance satellites watch for the movement of nuclear submarines from port and the dispersal of nuclear warheads from stockpiles. By gathering electronic intelligence, one side can even tap into the opponent's military warning network. When the North Koreans shot down an American EC-121 reconnaissance aircraft in 1969 in international airspace, President Nixon disclosed—presumably inadvertently—in a news conference that the United States was able to read Soviet radar and listen to Soviet military progress in tracking the aircraft.

The danger of this intimate reaction between the two command structures is that actions of one will be perceived and countered with stronger reactions by the other. In time of crisis, a small "signal" could rapidly reverberate, triggering increasingly significant responses and a war that neither side intended. Both sides are certainly aware that even the first stages of a nuclear alert, once undertaken, might prove irreversible. An advanced stage, such as the ordering of strategic bombers into the air to await further orders, would carry even higher risks. Since the founding of the Strategic Air Command, in 1946, there has never been a precautionary launch of American bombers. "During the past twenty years," notes Bracken, "both the United States and the Soviet Union have built highly interactive warning systems of incomprehensible complexity. With these systems tightly coupling the nuclear arsenals of each side, the effect of small perturbations is amplified throughout the entire nuclear force system."[15]

The two nuclear command structures by which each superpower controls its nuclear deterrent in fact constitute a single system. Each structure is tightly linked to the other by its monitoring of the other's actions and its propensity to respond to them. In peacetime the two systems act to suppress false alarms and disturbances and exert negative control. In time of crisis their behavior is the opposite. Then a trifling disturbance might lead to catastrophic failure, whatever the intent of political authorities.

3

Flash, Blast, and Fire

The First Minute

The explosion of a nuclear weapon is an event of immense power and, in an abstract sense, even beauty. Within a fraction of a millionth of a second, the nuclear materials and casing of a one-megaton weapon are transformed into a packet of energy five times hotter than the center of the sun.

Out of this mini-sun bursts a flash of X rays so intense that the air for several feet around the weapon is heated into an incandescent ball.

This little fireball, only a few millionths of a second old, contains the vaporized contents of the weapon, and a vast flux of energy created by the fission and fusion reactions of the nuclear explosion. So immense an amount of energy packed into a tiny space creates temperatures of 100 million degrees centigrade and pressures of millions of pounds per square inch. A violent expansion begins.

In less than a thousandth of a second, the fireball of a one-megaton weapon has grown to 440 feet across. In ten seconds, the fireball is more than a mile in diameter.[1]

Like the sun, the fireball radiates heat and light. But its brief life is more violent and more intense. Along with the initial pulse of light, a flux of radiation—neutrons and gamma rays—escapes from the weapon. Though the radiation carries away only 3 percent of the weapon's energy, it damages or destroys the body tissues of those within range. After the initial pulse of light, as the X rays burst out of the bomb casing, the ballooning fireball slows and cools to about 300,000 degrees. At this point, a shock wave of squeezed air starts to propagate ahead of it. The air is so compressed and heated that it becomes a luminous, glowing shell, two and a half times as bright as the sun's surface, but masking the even brighter fireball within it.

For a few thousandths of a second, the explosion consists of two concentric shells, the glowing shell of compressed air and, pushing behind it, the intenser shell of hot gases liberated by the nuclear explosion. Then, as the expanding outer shell cools to below 8,000 degrees, it becomes transparent again, and the full brightness of the fireball shines through.

In this second pulse of light, far brighter than the first, about a third of the weapon's energy is beamed away. To an observer nine miles away, the fireball would appear 100 times brighter than a desert sun at noon. The burst of heat and light, known as a thermal pulse, lasts for about ten seconds. The light is like the sun's but so intense that it kindles fires and burns exposed skin up to nine miles away.

Within a minute the fireball has cooled so much that it has ceased to glow. Meanwhile, a third effect of the weapon, more immediately deadly than the radiation and the double pulse of light, is continuing to develop. This is the shock wave created by the fireball's expansion. The wave is a hard wall of compressed air followed by roaring winds. Ten seconds after the explosion, when the fireball has reached its full size, the shock front is already some three miles ahead. Almost half the weapon's energy is transferred to the pounding wave.

When the shock wave reaches the ground, a secondary wave is generated by reflection, much as a sound wave produces an echo. The reflected wave joins the primary wave, increasing its strength, as both propagate outward along the ground. The height at which the bomb is detonated can be chosen so that this enhanced shock wave, known as a reinforced Mach front, produces the greatest possible area of destruction.

Consider a frame house four miles from ground zero, the point on the earth's surface right beneath the explosion. During the first ten seconds after detonation, radiant power from the thermal pulse arrives at such a rate that black smoke pours off the paint in front of the house. Inside the house, any materials in line of sight of the intense light explode into violent flames almost instantly.

The thermal pulse ceases, followed by a lull of five seconds. Then the shock wave arrives. It lasts for three seconds, 30 times as long as the blast from a nonnuclear bomb, and is followed by winds of more than 150 miles an hour. The shock wave strikes the house, then envelopes it with high pressure air and winds. The building is simultaneously knocked down and crushed as the shock wave rushes past.

The farther the shock wave travels, the more its forces ebb. After 40 seconds, the shock front from a one-megaton weapon has reached 10 miles from ground zero, and its pressure is only one pound per square inch greater than normal atmospheric pressure, but still enough to knock out windows and some doors. After 50 seconds, when the fireball is no longer visible, the shock wave has reached 12 miles from ground zero and has slowed to slightly faster than the speed of sound.

Within a minute of detonation the weapon has done its primary damage. If visibility is good, the thermal pulse has kindled numerous fires everywhere within 4 miles of ground zero and has set newspapers alight at even up to 12 miles. The shock wave has caused extremely severe damage within four miles of ground zero, with slowly diminishing levels of damage out to ten miles and beyond. The wave may have blown out some of the fires ignited by the thermal pulse but, by wrecking buildings and fuel tanks, it has opened up their contents to future attack by flames. The streets are blocked with debris, the water pressure drops to zero because of damaged and leaking pipes. The air is full of flying debris and window shards, much of it traveling at lethal velocities. Most people within five miles of ground zero have died of blast, with less and less mortality out to 12 miles. Some of the blast victims have ruptured lungs and abdomens pierced by debris, others have been hurled through the air and slammed into walls or surfaces with deadly force. Many people have sustained up to third-degree burns from the thermal pulse.

Now, one minute after detonation, everything is set for even greater damage to begin.

The Fire Storm

The fireball, a mass of superheated air, is far lighter than the atmosphere around it. Like a bubble of air in deep water, its buoyancy propels it upward. The fireball from a one-megaton bomb exploded a mile above a city shoots up 5 miles in a minute. As it rises, the fiery bubble expands and is squashed into a doughnut shape, forming the familiar mushroom cloud. In the wake of the bubble's ascent, rushing winds are drawn up carrying dirt and debris from the shattered city. The updraft, flowing through the middle of the doughnut and out and around its periphery, forms the stem of the mushroom. On the ground the updraft sucks cool air into and up the stem, creating massive winds rushing in toward ground zero. After ten minutes the mushroom cloud reaches its maximum height of 12 miles or so and begins to spread sideways until, after an hour, it is dispersed by winds and merges with the natural clouds in the sky.

Meanwhile, the outward winds created by the shock wave have started to reverse and rush inward, following the winds being drawn up the mushroom stem. The inward winds fan the fires set by the thermal pulse. The fires grow into conflagrations, spread at the direction of the winds. If there is enough combustible material and if enough fires are set simultaneously over a large area, the phenomenon known as a fire storm begins.

In a fire storm many fires merge to form a single column of hot gases rising from the burning area. Like the mushroom stem, the new, broader column sucks in winds that feed the fires. One effect of the inward-rushing winds is to keep the fire from spreading further, sharply defining its edge. The other effect is that, within the area of the fire storm, everything burnable is consumed.

Hiroshima and Nagasaki

These are the effects that it is thought will occur when a one-megaton weapon is exploded above a city. No such weapon has been used in this way. The bases of estimation are the two nuclear weapons dropped on Hiroshima and Nagasaki in August 1945, the test explosions conducted in the atmosphere until 1963, when testing of nuclear weapons above ground was renounced by treaty, and the massive incendiary raids conducted against German and Japanese cities in World War II.

The Hiroshima and Nagasaki weapons give only an approximate guide to the effects of modern warheads because they were so small. The yield of nuclear warheads is measured in terms of the tons of chemical explosive (TNT) that would be needed to produce the same effect. One megaton (1 million tons of TNT) is a yield in the mid-range of the strategic warheads in today's arsenals. Most Soviet warheads are considerably larger, most having yields of 1, 2, 15, or 25 megatons. American warheads, because they can be delivered more accurately, do not need so great a yield to destroy protected targets. Most have yields of 0.04, 0.17, 0.20, or 1.00 megatons.[2]

The nuclear weapons used against Japan in World War II were a fraction of the size of today's weapons. Little Boy, the bomb dropped on Hiroshima on 6 August 1945, had a yield of only 0.0125 megatons, or 12.5 kilotons. Fat Man, exploded over

Nagasaki on 9 August, was a 22.0 kiloton weapon. Yet the effect of these small devices on the cities was devastating.

The Hiroshima bomb was dropped from a height of 9,600 meters (31,500 feet) just past 8:15 in the morning. People were on their way to work, since an earlier air raid alert had been called off. Forty-three seconds later, at a height of about 580 meters, the weapon exploded.

At ground zero, the point immediately beneath the weapon, the temperature reached above 3,000 degrees centigrade. Half a mile from ground zero, the thermal pulse created temperatures of 1,800 degrees, making roof tiles bubble, charring trees and telephone poles, and setting paper and blackout curtains on fire.[3]

The blast wave from the weapon collapsed or greatly damaged all wooden buildings out to 2.5 miles from ground zero and seriously damaged concrete buildings within half this radius. The blast wave blew out or smothered some of the fires set by the thermal pulse but broke open the combustible contents of houses as tinder for other fires.

Many thousands were killed instantly by the thermal pulse, by radiation, or by the blast wave. Any one of these effects was probably lethal for those outside in the streets within 0.6 miles of ground zero. Even within the distance, however, some degree of protection against radiation and thermal burns was provided by wooden houses and more by concrete buildings.

In the central zone beneath the bomb, the thermal pulse burned clothes and burned and charred skin, often burning through to the viscera.

At greater distances the thermal pulse was more selective, burning through black clothes, which absorbed the light, but being reflected by white garments. Many victims received severe burns on exposed skin but were protected in parts that were clothed. Some even had the pattern of the clothing etched into the skin, the bomb light burning through dark parts of the pattern and being excluded by the lighter regions. Almost all caught out in the open within 1.1 miles of ground zero received fatal burns. Burns severe enough to need treatment were suffered as far away as 2.6 miles.

Many victims within the central zone were blown away by the blast and hurled with lethal force into the ground or buildings. Shards of flying glass from blast-shattered windows were a major hazard. "Injuries to blood vessels and peripheral nerves were caused by large flying fragments," reports the committee appointed by the cities of Hiroshima and Nagasaki to record the bomb damage. "Wounds from glass splinters were frequent and led to multiple small lacerations or to cut wounds with embedded splinters. Although these multiple wounds themselves were not fatal, they caused great pain and agony. With the fall of individual resistance following radiation injury, the wounds became infected and frequently led to gangrenous changes."

Besides breaking open the city for the ensuing flames, the blast wave also destroyed its capacity to fight fires. Most firefighting equipment was crushed in the collapse of the firehouse buildings. Only one fireman in five was able to respond for duty. Yet firemen found that, because of leaks and damage to pipes, the pressure in the water mains had dropped precipitously. Even if men and machines had survived the blast, they found that many streets were blocked by debris, making fires inaccessible.

Within 20 to 30 minutes after the explosion, a mass fire began, probably of the type known as a fire storm. Hiroshima is built on the delta of the Ota River, which flows into the Seto Inland Sea. The seven branches of the Ota divide the city into six islands. Though these should have served as firebreaks, so many fires had been lit simultaneously that the river had little retarding effect. With so many fires ablaze, cold air from outside was sucked in toward the burning area of the city from all directions, creating a fire storm. The wind grew steadily in force, reaching speeds of 30 to 40 miles an hour about two to three hours after the explosion, finally calming at about 5:00 P.M. Accompanying the fire was black rain, droplets of moisture laden with minute particles of carbon from the fire. The black rain, containing radioactivity from the explosion, fell intermittently on Hiroshima from 9:00 A.M. until 4:00 P.M.

Fed by oxygen from the inward-rushing winds, the fire storm burned so intensely that, within the burnout area of Hiroshima, everything combustible was consumed. An area of 4.4 square miles was reduced to waste and ashes. Only the gutted shells of concrete or iron-frame buildings remained standing.

Escape was difficult for all except those on the periphery of the burnout area. Very few survivors with concussion or serious limb injuries reached the hospitals; most were unable to escape the conflagration. Of those within 1,500 feet of ground zero, 88 percent were killed immediately or died the same day. Yet some survived even from this inner zone. One, Eizo Nomura, was in the Fuel Hall, a building almost directly beneath the explosion. The account of Nomura's escape illustrates many of the physical features that follow a nuclear explosion over a city.

At the moment of detonation, Nomura had gone to the basement of the building to search for a document. He and eight others escaped from the rubble of the building and struggled through flaming streets to some stone steps beside the Motoyasu River, one of the seven branches of the Ota. This is the account of his journey:

"His hair had all been burnt away, and his skin was so damaged that large areas of the flesh beneath lay exposed. Blood was oozing from the many wounds he had sustained on both face and body. His clothing hung in shreds. For a time, neither he nor his fellow workers uttered a word; like phantoms, they stared blankly ahead. But now that the flames around them had begun to spread, the gray cloud in which they had been immersed lifted somewhat. Feeling the growing heat on his own torn body, Nomura slithered two steps downward, closer to the river. Since the water seemed to be sinking, he descended one step more.

"All around him, flames leapt into the sky, and from the

burning buildings billowed great clouds of thick black smoke. Shards of red-hot metal and bits of burning wood rained down upon the nine people who had sought refuge beside the river. Their instinct was to look upward, in the hope of evading the fiery downpour; but when they did, they found that the billowing smoke was extremely painful to their already torched eyes. . . .

"Then great drops of rain began to fall; it was not like ordinary rain at all—it was dark and heavy and extremely cold. In no time at all, the nine men and women were drenched and chilled. Shivering, they mounted the steps and cautiously approached one of the blazing buildings. In about half an hour they began to feel somewhat warmer, and then they realized that they had better try to escape from the fiery inferno around them. They got as far as the Aioi Bridge, but the situation there was no better. The smoke from the burning buildings was so dense they could hardly see to move any further.

"Nomura decided, nonetheless, that he would try to get away and, if possible, find help for the others. . . . That walk through Hiroshima was like taking a stroll through the lowest reaches of hell. The whole city seemed to be on fire. Wherever he walked, clouds of stinking black smoke belched out at him. Dead bodies lay sprawled where they had fallen. Now and then a silent, ghostly figure would cross his path. All the people he saw were injured—burnt or bleeding or both—and all were nearly naked. Their clothing had been burned away or literally torn from their backs by the blast. . . . Only later did the realization come to him that he had been one of the few lucky ones."[4]

Another survivor from close in was a schoolgirl, Taeko Nakamae. With a score of girls from the city's high schools, she was working at the Central Telephone Exchange, a third of a mile from ground zero, when the weapon detonated. The roof of the building fell in, burying the girls in piles of debris. "Badly burned and badly injured, they began to cry out in the darkness. Suddenly they heard the shrill voice of their homeroom teacher,

Mrs. Wakita: 'Get up, all of you! Get up! We must fight on until the final victory!' "

With Mrs. Wakita's help, Taeko managed to extricate herself from the debris and leave through one of the windows. "Outside, she saw scorched trees, fallen telephone and electric poles, and collapsed houses, all licked by tongues of living flame. Joining a host of others, all as black as the scorched trees, she began to run in the direction of Mount Hiji, but after a little while she had to stop: she had no breath left. Numbly, she watched two children—a boy of about ten and a girl of six. 'Mako! Mako!' she heard the boy cry. 'Please don't die! Mako, are you dead?' The little girl made no reply. As Taeko watched, the weeping boy took the corpse of his little sister into his arms. No one else paid any attention to the scene. Flames were closing in; everyone in the area who could still move, however slowly or painfully, was trying to escape.

"Taeko moved on. At last she was in sight of Tsurami Bridge, beyond which lay Mount Hiji. As she approached, she saw a vast number of people sitting on the bridge. Most of them were completely naked; a few still wore shreds of tattered clothing. All were burnt. Their bodies were as black as though they had been coated with soot, except where patches of open wound showed red. With some, the skin of their backs had simply fallen away and flapped about in the wind like fluttering shirttails. Faces were swollen, with their features distorted beyond recognition. As Taeko stood there for a moment, she realized that the number of refugees fleeing from the stricken center of the city was growing ever greater.

"Among them she saw some of her fellow workers from the Telephone Exchange Bureau, as well as one of the department heads. Looking at Taeko, he said: 'You seem to be the worst hurt. We'll have to do something for you.' Taeko put her hands to her face, where she could feel blood oozing from the injuries; only then did she realize that she must be as disfigured as many of the others on the bridge. The department head took out a cigarette, crushed it, and pasted the tobacco over the worst of her wounds to staunch the flow of blood.

"The fires kept coming closer; the air was growing ominously hot; flames had already begun to lick at the bridge itself. To wait here any longer would be fatal. The bridge was crowded with refugees, tottering, creeping, or crawling across, impeded by the bodies of those who had already died.

" 'Let's try to swim across the river,' Taeko said to her little circle of friends from the bureau.

"They all nodded their agreement; but the tide from the Inland Sea was flowing in, and the river was deep and dangerous. Although Taeko was a good swimmer, one of the girls told her she ought not to try it because of her injuries. Mrs. Wakita, who had by now rejoined the group, said, 'Hold on to me—we'll get across the river together.'

"In midstream, however, Taeko's strength gave out. She could no longer move either arms or legs; she felt herself drifting into unconsciousness, and it seemed to her that she was already dead. But Mrs. Wakita was still holding onto her. 'Take courage, child,' she said. 'You can't die here.'

"Just then a boat approached the struggling girl and woman. A man's sturdy pair of arms reached down and helped to pull Taeko into the boat; Mrs. Wakita followed. When they reached the opposite bank, they carefully thanked their savior and then began to walk, with many others, toward a reception center. After they reached it, Mrs. Wakita murmured, 'Wait here just for a few minutes. I'll go and get the others.' . . .

"By that time it was mid-afternoon, and the remorseless August sun beat down onto the victims of the explosion who had taken refuge on Mount Hiji, at the eastern end of the city. One of these, Taeko Nakamae, overcome by all that had happened to her since 8:15 that morning, with the blistering sun now pouring relentlessly over her torn body, sank into merciful unconsciousness."[5]

Casualties at Hiroshima and Nagasaki

The toll of those killed at Hiroshima and Nagasaki is not precisely established, because both cities contained unknown numbers of soldiers and other transients in addition to their resident population. According to the joint commission appointed by the American and Japanese governments to investigate the effects of the bomb, 45,000 people died at Hiroshima on the day of bombing, and 91,000 were injured. Of the 91,000 living injured who survived the first day, 19,000 died later of their wounds, mostly within 20 days. The total of dead after four months was 64,000, with 72,000 surviving casualties. Only half the city's population—119,000 out of 255,000—escaped uninjured.[6]

These figures did not include military personnel, however. Nor does another tally compiled later by the Hiroshima City Survey Section, which almost doubles the number of dead. The city estimates that by 10 August 1946, a year after the bombing, 119,000 had died out of a population of 320,000. In addition, there were 80,000 surviving casualties, of whom 31,000 sustained severe injuries. Some 4,000 people were missing, and 119,000 were uninjured.[7]

The death toll at Nagasaki was smaller. Though the weapon used there had a slightly larger yield than that used in Hiroshima, the hilly terrain protected many inhabitants from direct flash injuries. Fires broke out about 90 minutes after the explosion, triggering a widespread conflagration. No definite fire storm occurred at Nagasaki, although a fierce wind blew whose velocity reached 35 miles an hour two hours after the explosion, tapering to 10 miles an hour seven hours later. But the wind blew the flames up a valley where there was nothing to burn. Black rain fell, as at Hiroshima. The area of total burnout was 1.1 square miles, a quarter of that at Hiroshima.

At Nagasaki, according to the joint commission, 22,000 people died on the day of the bombing, and another 17,000 afterward. There were 25,000 surviving casualties and 110,000 uninjured.[8] Higher figures are computed by the Nagasaki City Commission, which estimates that 74,000 had died by 31 December 1945 and that 75,000 were injured. It is not known whether these figures included the transient population of the city, such as soldiers and volunteers.

Of the injured in both cities, 70 percent suffered blast wounds, 65 percent had burns, from the thermal pulse or flames, and 30 percent suffered radiation injury. As the percentages show, many had multiple injuries.

The Use of Nuclear Weapons against Japan

The United States entered the First World War in large part because of revulsion at the German policy of unrestricted submarine warfare. Torpedoing merchant vessels and putting the lives of noncombatants at risk was specifically prohibited by the international agreement of 1930 between the United States, Britain, and Japan. Yet, by the end of the Second World War, American authorities had almost no hesitation in dropping nuclear weapons on the civilian inhabitants—men, women, and children—of Hiroshima and Nagasaki. Seldom since the Mongol invasions has the wholesale massacre of innocents been a deliberate element of warfare. But the United States and Britain, provoked by their opponents' unscrupulous attitude toward civilians, conducted numerous incendiary raids on German and Japanese cities during the Second World War. Because of that precedent, it is now taken for granted that only self-interest would prevent the combatants in a nuclear war from targeting their opponents' cities.

The Allies' incendiary raids not only provided a moral precedent for the use of nuclear bombs against cities but also matched them in destructiveness. Recently these incendiary bomb attacks have been restudied because of the unique information they provide about the likely effects of nuclear weapons on cities. As the Allies perfected their incendiary raids, they found that the largest fires were created when conventional bombs were used to break open buildings and incendiaries were then used to set them ablaze. The incendiaries had to fall within a small area so that separate fires could coalesce into a single mass fire. A nuclear weapon is the ideal incendiary device. Its thermal pulse sets buildings alight, and its blast wave crushes them into matchwood.

The moral path to the use of nuclear weapons in the Second World War led directly from the failure of conventional bombing. Britain's Royal Air Force started the war with the aim of destroying industrial targets essential to the German economy. That meant flying in daylight so that the pilots could see the targets. But the British bombers suffered an unendurable level of attrition from fighters and anti-aircraft guns, and the RAF switched to flying at night. In the darkness, though, the pilots could barely find the right city, let alone a particular factory. So they began to bomb the only targets they could safely hit—cities. The rationalization of the policy was that the target was German morale, to be destroyed by massive bombing of people's homes and workplaces. The means were successful, but the policy was a failure. Nearly one-fifth of Germany's houses were destroyed or heavily damaged. Some 300,000 civilians were killed and 780,000 wounded. The effect on the German economy was virtually nil.[9]

In the Pacific war against Japan, the U.S. Air Force was driven to the same goal, also by the failure of precision bombing. When island bases within range of Japan were captured in 1944, a series of raids was launched to cripple Japan's aircraft production. Because of high winds and frequent cloud cover, the pilots were able to do little damage. The head of the 21st Bomber Command, a longtime advocate of precision strategic bombing, was removed and replaced by a veteran of the bombing campaign against Germany, Major General Curtis LeMay. After two practice raids, LeMay on the night of 9 March 1945 launched a force of 334 bombers armed solely with incendiaries. Their target was a rectangular area of Tokyo. A large section of the city, with its wood and paper houses, was soon in flames. Its fire departments were poorly trained and equipped. The fires soon raged out of control. Entire block fronts burst into flame. In the canals water boiled. Clouds of smoke and soot filled the night sky. Almost 16 square miles of the city were burned out. Some 267,000 buildings were destroyed. Charred bodies were found afterward piled in heaps on bridges, roads, and canals. More than 83,000 people perished, and 41,000 were injured. The attack was the most destructive single bombing raid in history.[10]

LeMay was quick to follow up this success. By June 1945 he had devastated the six most important industrial cities of Japan —Tokyo, Nagoya, Kobe, Osaka, Yokohama, and Kawasaki, gutting over 40 percent of their urban areas and rendering millions homeless. He then attacked more than 50 smaller cities and industrial centers.

The Manhattan Project to develop the nuclear bomb was mounted because of strong evidence that German scientists understood the principles of nuclear fission and were working at Hitler's orders to develop a weapon. When Germany surrendered, on 7 May 1945, the formal reason for the Manhattan Project was no longer valid. Nevertheless, the project was so near fruition, the technical challenge held such fascination, that few scientists or officials harbored any serious thought of discontinuing their work. One physicist, Joseph Rotblat of the University of London, resigned, but others refused to let Germany's defeat distract them from completing the novel weapon they had come so close to creating.

The first atomic bomb was exploded at a test site in the New Mexico desert on the evening of 16 July 1945. The decision of President Truman and his advisers to use the new weapons on Japan was not unanimous. General Dwight Eisenhower, the Supreme Commander of Allied forces in Europe, urged that the weapon not be used, because Japan was almost defeated already and "because I thought that our country should avoid shocking world opinion by the use of [atomic weapons]."[11] But the incendiary raids, already an established instrument of Allied policy, had broken the moral barrier against the mass killing of civilians. "There was never any doubt that the bomb would be used," concludes the historian Ronald Spector. "Years of American talk about the Japanese as savage fanatics who cared nothing about human life had prepared the way for such a decision. The 'sneak attack' on Pearl Harbor, accounts of Japanese atrocities in prisoner of war camps and in occupied Asia, the kamikazes, and the bloody last-ditch resistance on Iwo Jima and Okinawa had confirmed and hardened these beliefs. 'When you deal with a beast you have to treat him as a beast,' wrote Truman a few days after Nagasaki."[12]

The Nature of Fire Storms

The nuclear weapons dropped on Hiroshima and Nagasaki initiated a vastly different form of war, yet in terms of pure physical destruction there was an unbroken continuum with the mass use of napalm-charged incendiary bombs against other cities. The Hiroshima bomb killed from 64,000 to 119,000 people; the March 9 raid on Tokyo killed 83,000. Incendiaries and nuclear weapons differ in many of their effects. The most destructive, which they hold in common, is the phenomenon of fire storms.

A fire storm is created when many individual fires coalesce into a mass fire and the columns of hot rising gases from each fire merge into a single mass column of heated air. Unlike conflagrations, in which the fire front is driven forward by prevailing winds, fire storms create their own dynamics. Once a fire storm is established, it ceases to spread, because the massive merged column of heated air sucks in air at ground level from all sides. Within the fire zone, the winds intensify the fire by fanning the flames and bringing fresh oxygen for combustion. Within the zone of the fire storm, such extreme temperatures are generated that nothing combustible is left unburned.

The record of previous large urban fires in history shows that the number of casualties depends on the speed with which the fire develops. The great fire of London in 1666 destroyed an area of almost a square mile but killed only 8 people, because it moved slowly. The fire that followed the San Francisco earthquake of 1906 spread from more than 30 separate ignitions and left 100,000 people homeless, but it, too, moved slowly enough to allow most of the population to escape; only 452 people perished. The first known fire storm seems to have arisen in 1934 at Hakodate, in Japan; 2,000 people died. But it was not until the incendiary raids of World War II that fire storms were recognized as a special phenomenon, as a result of the massive incendiary raids against German and Japanese cities.

Although incendiary raids were launched on 71 German and about 65 Japanese cities, fire storms were started on only a few occasions, when conditions were right. In Dresden the high, closely spaced buildings were laden with combustibles. The lack of an effective air defense allowed the British air force to concentrate its bombing, leading to many simultaneous fires. At least 135,000, and perhaps as many as 250,000, people died. Fire storms were also started in Hamburg, Kassel, Heilbronn, and Brunswick. Berlin was repeatedly firebombed, but its defenses prevented concentrated attacks, and the fires that were ignited never coalesced into the inferno of a fire storm.

The best-documented incendiary fire storm, and the one that probably most resembles what a nuclear weapon would do an American city, is one that occurred in the German city of Hamburg in July 1943.

The Allies mounted three massive incendiary raids on Hamburg. The first, on 24/25 July 1943, destroyed about one and a half square miles of the city. The second, on 27/28 July, burned five to six square miles in a fire storm. The third, on 29/30 July, involved about two square miles. Each raid was carried out by 700 planes, delivering about 1,300 tons of high explosive bombs, 500 tons of oil incendiaries, and 600 tons of magnesium incendiaries.

The incendiary bombs were designed to penetrate roofs and floors and settle into the interior of buildings, where tests had shown that fires were most efficiently set. The high explosive bombs, dropped at regular intervals so as to keep fire fighters in their shelters, were intended to block roads with rubble and craters.

In the second Hamburg raid, two out of every three buildings in the target area were ablaze within about 20 minutes. As the fires grew, sparks reached tinder in neighboring buildings through shattered windows. For three hours the fires intensified, then raged at full fury for another three.

During the period of intensification a hurricane of fire developed, accompanied by sporadic squalls, perhaps caused by the winds that were drawn into the fire from all directions. The rapid shift of the winds thwarted repeated attempts to establish firebreaks. At the edge of the fire, the winds were strong enough to uproot trees three feet in diameter and to prevent firemen from coming within hose range. Even the pilots of the bombers above the fire encountered hazardous turbulence from the heated air of the stricken city.

On the ground the burgeoning winds and fire soon made buildings crumble into the streets, trapping people and the firefighting units trying to save them. With many large fires raging unchecked, streets acted as channels for the fast winds flowing toward the center, and became filled with flames. Because of the searing heat and flying embers, even open spaces like parks could not be used as sanctuaries by the fire fighters.

The population of Hamburg had received adequate warning of the raid. Even so, thousands died in the streets. Yet those in the shelters were not better off. As the fires grew hotter, the heat and smoke in the shelters became intense. The occupants had to choose between the increasingly threatening conditions in the shelter, and the hurricane of fire in the streets. For most, escape was impossible. The area engulfed with fire was so large that the journey to the perimeter was too long.

Even for people in shelters close to the edge of the fire zone, escape was impossible. Those outside the zone saw hundreds of people leave the shelters, then slowly collapse from the heat after a few paces in the open, as if exhausted. Some tried to get up and continue. Others were engulfed in tornado-like fire whirls that propagated erratically down streets. Many caught in the fire whirls had their clothes burst into flames and died naked.

Those who stayed in the shelters faced a different end. As buildings collapsed under the heat and winds, many shelters were buried in debris. For some occupants, death came easily; as carbon monoxide seeped in, people slipped calmly into unconsciousness. In other shelters, rescuers found evidence of panic and attempts to escape.

The rubble became so hot that it was impossible to enter the area for two days after the raid. As late as 25 August, a month after the raid, it was still necessary to hose down the hot rubble and smoldering fires. Many of the buried shelters developed such intense heat from the overburden of hot rubble that excavators found shrunken bodies, often lying in a thick, greasy mass, which appeared to be melted body fat. Some bodies were reduced entirely to ash, and many of the shrunken bodies burned to ash within a few weeks of exposure to the air.

According to the reports of the German Fire Protection Police, 50,000 to 60,000 people were killed in the fire zone. There is no clear evidence as to how many people, if any, were rescued from the firestorm zone. At the peak of the fire's intensity, five to six square miles were simultaneously in flames. The power output probably reached one or two million megawatts.

In all firebombed cities surveyed by German medical teams, carbon monoxide poisoning was regarded as the primary cause of death, accounting for up to 80 percent of all casualties. Blast was a quite rare cause of death, affecting only those within about 27 yards of the explosions.

Nuclear Weapons and Fire Storms

To reach a better understanding of fire storms, H. L. Brode and R. D. Small of the Pacific-Sierra Research Corporation have developed a computer-run mathematical model that explains many of the features observed in historical fire storms.[13] Their calculations show that throughout the fire zones the average ground-level air temperatures in a fire storm are higher than the boiling point of water. For those who survived the initial radiation, thermal pulse, and blast of a nuclear explosion, the fire storm and its heat would pose an extremely hostile environment.

Large-scale fires, according to the computer models, generate hurricane-force winds, approaching 90 miles per hour, with velocities in streets or channels being even higher. The induced fire winds are drawn into the burning city from far away, their speed being noticeable up to 25 miles from the fire's edge. The inflow feeds the fire with oxygen and is turned upward into a broad smoke column. The soot from the fire may be carried high by the rising winds, but its ascent, according to the computer model, is effectively capped by the tropopause, the boundary between the lower and upper atmosphere.

For survivors of the nuclear blast and thermal pulse, a very significant feature of superfires is the noxious gases they generate. Among the most abundant are carbon dioxide and carbon monoxide. These act in fatal synergism. Carbon dioxide, the waste gas breathed out from the lungs, is also the body's physiological signal to start breathing faster. A higher level of carbon dioxide in the bloodstream initiates the extra breathing that dispels it. Carbon monoxide is a deadly gas because it displaces oxygen on the hemoglobin in red blood cells. As the burden of carbon monoxide grows, the body's tissues are starved of oxygen. Survivors exposed to high levels of both gases are forced to breath harder by the carbon dioxide, and thus to absorb all the more carbon monoxide and other noxious gases.

Heat also increases the breathing rate. Even if not fatal by itself—several hours' exposure to air temperatures much above 130 degrees Fahrenheit is usually fatal—heat can quickly worsen the effects of carbon dioxide and carbon monoxide. Other noxious gases likely to spew from burning materials are sulfur dioxide, nitrogen dioxide, and hydrogen cyanide.

Survivors within the fire zone of an attacked city would face a combination of high heat, noxious gases, smoke, and the physiological stresses of fear and hysteria. People in shelters would face a similar predicament unless the shelter had been specially designed to exclude heat and gases. This would require deep bunkers with their own generators and bottled air—the kind of refuge likely to be available only for top government leaders.

Another hazard for those in and around the firezone would be the toxic combustion products of the many chemicals and petroleum products stored in modern cities. Hydrogen chloride, hydrogen cyanide, sulfur dioxide, and phosgene are among the poisonous gases likely to be created in the fires. The hazardous chemicals known as dioxins might be created from combustion of the polychlorinated biphenyl compounds (PCBs) used in insulators. Clouds of asbestos fibers would be released from shattered buildings. All these substances would add to the perils of those who survived the direct effects of a nuclear weapon and its ensuing fire storm.[14]

Portrait of a One-Megaton Explosion

A nuclear weapon is a highly efficient incendiary, since it sets many fires simultaneously over a large area. On a clear day, with good visibility and no clouds to impede the light, a nuclear weapon with explosive power equivalent to one megaton of TNT would set fires over a wide area of a city. A reasonable estimate is that that area would be a circle of about seven and a half miles in radius from ground zero. The thermal pulse at this distance would deliver heat of ten calories per square centimeter, enough to ignite light fabrics, curtains, and other combustible materials. Heavy fog or clouds would shrink the area of thermal fires; dry summer weather would increase it. If the attack occurred when there was snow on the ground, the snow would reflect the thermal pulse into the interior of houses, kindling extra fires.

When a one-megaton weapon is exploded at the most effective height, the blast wave at seven and a half miles from ground zero exerts about two pounds per square inch above the normal pressure of the atmosphere. This is strong enough to shatter windows, blow out doors, and knock down interior walls that don't carry a building's load. Buildings damaged this way become well-aired structures, ideal for promoting any fires that develop. The blast wave would probably start quite a few fires, even at this distance, by overturning stoves, breaking gas lines, and shorting out electrical circuits.

Thus, over an area of 175 square miles, numerous simultaneous fires could develop. The precise area is of course highly uncertain, for it depends on the weather conditions, the local geography, and the combustible materials in the city. The height at which the bomb explodes also matters. A high altitude explosion could burn a city even though only a small blast wave would reach it. A surface burst, one whose fireball touches the ground, radiates only half as much heat as an airburst. Civil defense preparations could make a considerable difference at the edges of fires, but most passive measures are of limited value. Clearing land to make firebreaks would be of little help if fires started on both sides or burning firebrands were blown across. Removing all vehicles and their flammable fuel tanks would help, but short of tearing down a city, it would be hard to reduce significantly its propensity to burn. Active fire fighting during or after a nuclear attack would probably be quite impractical, because of the overwhelming number of fires and the blocking of roads by debris.

As the individual fires burn and gather strength, each heats the surrounding air, and the heated volumes of air expand and rise. If enough combustible material is present, the heat becomes sufficiently intense to generate the areawide air motion that gathers into a fire storm. Each layer of air above the smoldering city is pushed to a higher level, creating a broad ascending column. Cold air rushes into the city from all sides, bringing fresh oxygen to the fires. The process feeds on itself, the fire winds fanning the individual fires and spreading firebrands to kindle others. A fire of gigantic scale and ferocity can develop, with hurricane-force ground winds and temperatures that cause combustible materials to ignite spontaneously. The circulating system that causes the fire storm can grow to 9 miles in radius, according to the computer model of Brode and Small. In a multiple attack, fire storms whose centers are less than 18 miles or so apart could merge, greatly increasing the area of conflagration.

The fire storm created by a one-megaton nuclear weapon exploded over a typical urban area in the United States would probably build up so quickly that only those in the outer edge of the fire zone would have time to escape.

Death from Superfires

How many casualties is a one-megaton weapon likely to cause? In estimating the deaths and injuries sustained in hypothetical nuclear attacks, government agencies take the effects of blast at Hiroshima as a standard measure. Knowing the numbers killed and injured there at each level of blast, it is easy to calculate how many would be killed or injured by the greater blast of a one-megaton or larger-yield weapon. Blast is used as the main index because injuries from thermal effects are influenced by unpredictable factors like the degree of shielding; also, at Hiroshima, the destructive effects of the thermal pulse diminished with distance at very much the same rate as did the force of the blast wave.

But the blast method may be an inaccurate way to estimate the effects of larger weapons. The reason is that the effects of the thermal pulse from a one-megaton weapon drop off far more slowly with distance than does the blast wave. Hence the fires set by the thermal pulse, and the superfires that ensue, may kill people throughout an area considerably greater than the area in which blast alone causes death.

Many who would be counted as unharmed or injured under the blast methodology would be killed in the superfire, according to new calculations by Theodore Postol of Stanford University.[15] The radius of a superfire from ground zero would be heavily influenced by local conditions, such as atmospheric visibility and the nature and distribution of combustible materials in the city. In ordinary conditions a superfire might range out to seven and a half miles from ground zero. But if there were snow on the ground, to reflect the light of the thermal pulse into buildings, or cloud cover to reflect it back to earth, the superfire might range out to ten miles.

Within a superfire the near hurricane force winds and temperatures above that of boiling water would probably make survival impossible. Assuming a superfire radius of seven and a half miles, within which everyone dies, and the usual deaths and injuries from blast beyond that radius, Postol calculates that fatalities caused by superfires might be two to four times greater than those predicted by government agency estimates, based on blast alone. There would be far fewer injured survivors than the blast method projects, since many of these are considered fatalities under the superfire method. This is consistent with the findings of German and American reviews of the incendiary raids of World War II; the ratio of deaths to injured was much higher when incendiaries, rather than high explosives, were the major source of damage from air raids.

The effects of superfires were widely recognized at the end of World War II but have since been studied by only a small group of researchers. Strategic planners and decision makers may have poor understanding of their effects, and hence of the full consequences of nuclear weapons. Lack of such understanding can only increase the possibility of misjudgment and miscalculation.

4

Fallout

Perhaps the most feared aftereffect of nuclear weapons is radioactive fallout. Radiation cannot be sensed, except for a tingling sensation caused by very intense doses. Massive doses may be fatal immediately or within a few hours. Large doses cause radiation sickness, from which victims may take days or weeks to die. Those who survive lesser amounts face an extra risk of cancer in the years ahead. Even the fallout released in a single nuclear reactor accident, such as the explosion in April 1986 at the Chernobyl reactor in the Soviet Union, can expose hundreds of thousands of people to medically significant amounts of radiation.

The initial radiation created by a nuclear weapon is a relatively minor factor in mortality since two other effects—blast and heat—kill and destroy over a wider area. Radioactive fallout, however, can be lethal over a far larger area than all three. Fallout began to be studied seriously only after a test explosion at Bikini Atoll in the Pacific in 1954, when an unexpected change of wind carried hazardous levels of radiation over inhabited islands. The precise pattern of fallout likely to be created by a nuclear explosion depends heavily on the height of the burst and on the pattern of prevailing winds. For lack of sufficient evidence, the vulnerability of the human body to radiation is a matter of debate and continuing research.

Airbursts and Surface Bursts

A nuclear explosion is caused by the intense flux of radiation —neutrons and gamma rays—emitted from the nuclear materials. Much of the radiation is absorbed in the bomb debris and surrounding air, making them intensely radioactive. These radioactive materials, and the substances (known as fission products) into which the uranium and plutonium atoms break down, start to release radiation instantly. The process of radiation release, known as radioactive decay, may continue for days or years, depending on the nature of the radioactive element, and lasts until the radioactive atoms have turned into stable or nonradioactive forms.

The radiation from nuclear weapons is usually considered in two parts, "initial" and "residual." Initial radiation is defined as that produced during the first minute after detonation. It consists of the neutrons and gamma rays that escape directly from the nuclear reaction, and of the radiation emitted from the newly created radioactive materials. After a minute a nuclear fireball of almost any yield will have risen so high that its radiation no longer reaches the ground.[1] The longer the materials carrying the residual radiation stay airborne, the more they will decay toward harmless levels. But sooner or later the radioactive materials will fall or be washed out of the sky as fallout.

At Hiroshima and Nagasaki many were killed or injured by the initial radiation. Apart from the "black rain" that fell the day of the explosion, fallout from the two weapons was probably insignificant and, in any case, not measured. With modern weapons the effect would probably be the reverse. Initial radiation would be of little significance, because everyone within lethal range would also be within the lethal range of the thermal pulse and the blast wave.

Residual radiation is likely to be a significant feature of any future nuclear exchange because many weapons are likely to be detonated at or near ground level. Surface bursts, as they are termed, might be chosen for attacks against specially protected or "hardened" targets like missile silos. Unlike airbursts, surface bursts vaporize vast quantities of soil or rock, which are sucked into the fireball and become radioactive by mixing with the radioactive remnants of the bomb. Depending on the prevailing winds, the copious amounts of radioactive material so created can contaminate vast areas with lethal levels of radioactivity.

The full danger of fallout began to be appreciated after the United States exploded a 15-megaton weapon at Bikini Atoll, in the Pacific, on 1 March 1954. The device was detonated seven feet above the surface of a coral reef and is probably the nearest known approximation to what a surface burst nuclear weapon would be like. Code-named Bravo, the device contaminated an area of about 7,000 square miles with lethal amounts of radioactive fallout. Lesser levels of fallout covered a larger, teardrop-shaped area extending 330 statute miles downwind of the atoll and up to 60 miles wide. People on Rongelap Island and Alinginae Atoll, downwind of Bikini, were evacuated after two days, by which time some 267 had received heavy doses of up to 175 rads, more than a third of the lethal dose.* The uninhabited northern tip of Rongelap, 100 miles downwind of the explosion, received 3,300 rads in the four days following the test.[2]

Some of the Marshall Islanders suffered delayed effects, such as thyroid gland abnormalities that started to appear nine years after the blast. Worse affected was the crew of a Japanese tuna-fishing boat, the *Fukuryu Maru No. 5* (Lucky Dragon No. 5),

---

*A rad is one of the units used to measure ionizing radiation absorbed by the body. Ionizing radiation includes X rays, electrons, and neutrons that are energetic enough to create charged particles (ions) by stripping electrons away from atoms as they pass through matter. One rad represents the absorption of a certain amount of ionizing radiation—specifically, the absorption of 100 ergs of ionizing radiation per gram of body tissue.

operating 100 miles east of Bikini. The white limestone ashes from the vaporized coral reef rained down on the boat for six hours, and the crew soon started to complain of headaches and nausea. When the boat returned to its home port of Yaizu 13 days later, all 23 members of the crew were diagnosed as suffering from radiation-caused symptoms, such as blisters and loss of hair. One of the crewmen died six months later.[3]

What levels of radioactive fallout might be expected from a nuclear exchange between the superpowers? How much land would be contaminated and for how long? The best available answers are guesses based on the above-ground nuclear tests like Bravo that were conducted before the 1963 treaty that banned tests in the atmosphere. The estimates are further limited by the many factors that affect fallout, from weather conditions to the form of the nuclear attack.

The yield of the warheads in both American and Soviet arsenals has tended to diminish as missiles have grown more accurate and the destruction of targets can be assured with smaller weapons. Small nuclear weapons, paradoxically, can create more fallout than larger weapons, because the fireball rises less high in the atmosphere and the fallout comes down sooner, with less time to decay.

Nuclear weapons that work on the principle of fission—atoms splitting apart to release energy—create considerably more radioactivity than do weapons that work purely by fusion—atoms fusing together to release energy. In practice, fusion weapons have a fission weapon as their trigger. Most warheads are generally assumed to be fission-fusion hybrids.

Fallout also depends on the particles that are sucked up into the fireball and on the height to which they are carried. The largest particles fall out first under their own weight. Those falling out within 24 hours of the explosion are defined as "local" fallout, because they are deposited at or downwind of ground zero. The smaller particles, known as "global" fallout, may stay aloft for weeks or months and settle far from their origin. Global fallout is considerably less harmful than local fallout because it is far more dispersed and has longer to decay.

The pattern of local fallout depends on the prevailing winds. If these blow steadily, fallout will be spread in an elongated, cigar-shaped pattern downwind of ground zero, with radioactivity being highest down the center of the cigar and lowest at the far end and edges. More often, winds shift, or blow from different directions at different heights, leading to a more complex pattern of fallout.

If all the radioactivity from a one-megaton, all-fission weapon were to arrive on the ground within an hour of detonation and to be evenly spread so as give a lethal dose (450 rads within 48 hours), it would cover an area of 15,500 square miles. In reality, because much of the radioactivity stays airborne longer and the local fallout is not evenly distributed, the area of lethal contamination from such a weapon is expected to measure only about 400 square miles. A 50 percent fission weapon would contaminate an area half this size.

The 450 rads with which the area is contaminated is the currently accepted value for the LD-50/60—the dose that would kill half the people exposed within 60 days, assuming that they were in no way shielded from it. The inside of a building offers a little shielding, a basement somewhat more, and specially constructed shelters afford considerable protection. Clean-up measures, such as removal of contaminated soil, can reduce radioactivity. So can the runoff after a rainfall. And the body's ability to repair radiation damage means that a dose that would be lethal if it arrived all at once can be better tolerated if spread out over a longer period.

In a major nuclear exchange thousands of warheads could be detonated. A calculation of the area of radioactive fallout depends heavily on how much the fallout patterns of individual weapons overlap, as would, for example, those of the many warheads likely to be aimed at Minuteman missile fields. In a worst-case analysis of 1982, T. F. Harvey of the Lawrence

Livermore National Laboratory assumed that each of 1,000 American cities was attacked with a one-megaton, 50 percent fission weapon that was detonated at surface level. His computer model indicated that 20 percent of the land area of the United States would be covered with lethal radiation. In part because of westerly winds, the radiation would be unevenly distributed, covering almost all the Northeast, half of the area east of the Mississippi, and only 10 percent west of it.

Another war scenario modeled by Livermore scientists assumes that 6,000 weapons of various yields, all 50 percent fission and 2,500 surface bursts, are fired at military and industrial targets in America, the Soviet Union, and European members of the NATO and Warsaw pacts. The computer predicts that the following land areas would be covered with lethal radiation: Europe, 3.2 percent; western Soviet Union, 3.8 percent; eastern Soviet Union, 5.3 percent; western United States, 6.0 percent; eastern United States, 5.3 percent.[4]

There are important qualifications to this overall calculation. It does not take account of the protective effects of buildings, so the 450-rad zone would be less lethal than otherwise; without shielding, half of those exposed to such a dose would die. Local geographical and weather conditions would make the fallout pattern more irregular than predicted by the computer, giving some hot spot areas more than the lethal dose and so reducing the overall lethal area. On the other hand, besides the lethal zone a much larger area would receive seriously debilitating doses of radiation (200 rads or more). Also the computer model takes account only of strategic nuclear weapons; tactical weapons, with smaller warheads, might well be used in Europe, increasing lethal fallout areas there by about 20 percent.

Global Fallout

Radiation from global fallout is a considerably less serious hazard in terms of immediate health effects. The radioactive particles have time to decay while airborne and are strewn far and wide when they descend. Instead of spreading intense radiation around and downwind of the explosion site, global fallout presents a different hazard—a low-level dose that continues over many years. These long-lasting low doses may increase the background rate of cancer.

Estimates of the global fallout from a large nuclear exchange have been rising. Ten years ago, global fallout in the Northern Hemisphere was predicted to amount to about 3 rads over 50 years; now the estimate is 30 rads over 50 years. The main reason for the increase is the trend toward smaller-yield weapons, the radioactivity of which is deposited lower in the atmosphere and descends hotter and sooner.

The lowermost part of the atmosphere, known as the troposphere, is the region in which all visible weather processes take place. Only when radioactive particles are in the troposphere can they be washed down by rain or snow. Above the troposphere is the stratosphere, where there is no rain. Particles in the stratosphere descend only because of gravity. Their settling rates can be very slow until they reach the troposphere and are rained out. Smaller weapons inject most of their radioactivity into the troposphere, from which it takes about a month to fall out. Larger weapons loft a larger share into the stratosphere, from which particles may take months or years to descend.

Scientists at the Lawrence Livermore National Laboratory have developed a computer model, named Glodep 2, that can be used to predict the global fallout rate, at various latitudes, that would result from a given scenario of nuclear war. For a large winter war in which weapons totaling 5,300 megatons in yield

are exploded, the model predicts 27 rads over 50 years for the
latitude band 30 to 50 degrees north, which includes the continental United States. Most of the radiation falls in the first
season after the war; progressively smaller amounts fall thereafter. If the war starts in the Northern Hemisphere's summertime, the fallout will total 21 rads instead of 27, because there
is less rain in summer to wash it down. The global fallout dose
per person is 12 rads for a summer war, 15 rads for a winter
war.

If the number of weapons were doubled, but each carried a
smaller warhead so as to keep the total megatonnage at 5,300,
the global fallout per person would increase to 27 rads over 50
years. By themselves, these low doses would probably not produce any immediate health effect. But, as discussed below, they
could cause a slight increase in the natural rate of cancer.
Though the increase would be very small, many millions of
people would be exposed to the enhanced global fallout, and the
number of extra cancer cases could be very large.

A major but only recently recognized consequence of nuclear
war is the effect of smoke and soot from burning cities on the
world's climate. How might the soot clouds, and the changed
structure of the stratosphere, affect the pattern of global fallout?
The present answer seems to be: not much. Using another computer model, and assuming that 150 million tons of smoke are
generated in a 5,300-megaton exchange, Livermore scientists
calculate that the average global fallout level would be reduced
by about 15 percent. This is much as would be expected, since
nuclear winter would reduce precipitation and hence retard the
deposition of fallout.

Targeting Nuclear Reactors

In a nuclear exchange an opponent might seek to destroy targets of industrial value, including power plants. A nuclear power plant could be put out of action by an airburst. But the possibility is sometimes raised that an opponent might target nuclear plants with surface bursts, so as to vaporize their nuclear components and contaminate a vast area with radioactivity. Many experts consider this an unlikely use of warheads. But what if it were to happen?

There are two elements to consider—the active nuclear fuel rods in the reactor's core and the spent rods that have been removed from the core. Since a national repository for long-term radioactive waste has not yet been established, and since there is no market demand for reprocessing used nuclear fuel, most nuclear power plants are putting their spent rods in nearby storage pools. These contain a vast amount of highly radioactive fission products from the breakdown of uranium fuel. A surface burst would certainly vaporize the storage pool and its contents.

Whether it would do the same to the active rods is less certain. Nuclear reactor cores are usually surrounded by a reinforced concrete building with walls a yard thick and a thick inner steel lining. The containment vessel inside the building is about four inches thick, and both the fuel rods and the cladding that protects them are designed to withstand high temperatures and pressures. All these barriers must be totally breached for the fuel's radioactivity to be spread in fallout like the weapon's. Only if a targeted reactor were included within a weapon's fireball is it probable that the core could contribute to local and global fallout.

Civilian reactors aside, those that power nuclear aircraft carriers and submarines would certainly be targets. Ships' reactors produce less power than commercial reactors, but a large ship with two reactors, designed to be used for many years without refueling, can contain nearly as much radioactivity as an operating commercial reactor.

Assuming the worst case, that reactors are targeted with surface bursts and hit so accurately that all their radioactivity is lofted into the air, even their short-term radiation would be greater than that of the one-megaton weapon that hit them, and their stored long-lived radioactivity very much larger. On the other hand, there are only 100 or so nuclear power plants at present operating in the United States, compared with the thousands of other major targets in a nuclear war. Thus the overall contribution of nuclear plants to the local fallout received in the first two days would probably add less than 10 percent to the total fallout at other targets.

Nuclear reactors would make a larger contribution to the global fallout because most of their radioactivity is in the form of radioactive elements with long lives. The worst case would be if one-megaton warheads were surface burst on 100 reactors and their spent fuel rod storage pools. Assume, too, that one fuel reprocessing plant were targeted, along with all the spent fuel rods it might be processing. Using the Glodep 2 computer model again and assuming a 5,300-megaton nuclear exchange, the total global fallout adds up to 95 rads over 50 years in the latitude band between 30 and 50 degrees north. Of the 95 rads, 33 are contributed by the weapons alone, 9 by the nuclear reactors and their active fuel rods, 33 by their spent fuel rods, and 20 by the single reprocessing plant.

If nuclear power plants and fuel reprocessing facilities in every country in the world were attacked, the above contributions to global fallout would be three times as great, according to the Glodep 2 model.[5]

These levels of global fallout would cause a slight increase in the cancer rate among populations exposed to them. Local fallout remains the prime danger of nuclear weapons.

The Lessons of Chernobyl

The reach of global fallout was vividly demonstrated by the accident that occurred on 26 April 1986 at the Soviet Chernobyl nuclear reactor at Pripyat, in the Ukraine. A significant portion of the radioactivity in the reactor was ejected into the atmosphere following an explosion and fierce fire in the reactor's graphite core. The fallout quickly spread throughout the Northern Hemisphere, exposing hundred of thousands of Russians and Eastern Europeans to medically significant quantities of radiation.

Soviet authorities have said the accident occurred at a time when the reactor was operating at low power. The power suddenly rose, apparently in connection with an experiment being conducted then, and the massive heat surge led to an explosion that blew through the reactor ceiling and ignited a fire in the graphite core.

At the time the Soviet Union said nothing about the incident, the worst in the history of nuclear power. But two days later, on 28 April, radioactivity twice the normal background level was detected at the Studsvik monitoring station in Sweden. In small areas north of Stockholm, where the radioactivity was washed down by rain, the dose rate increased to up to one millirem per hour, or 100 times the normal rate. The samples measured in Sweden contained radioactive iodine and cesium, elements that are easily vaporized. More surprisingly, they also contained less volatile elements, a sign that very high temperatures had been reached in the reactor core and that there had been no effective barrier to retain these elements.[6]

Working from the Swedish data, which suggested the Chernobyl reactor had been in operation for about 400 days, Joseph Knox of the Lawrence Livermore Radiation Laboratory calculated that the reactor had accumulated an inventory of 80 million curies of iodine-131 and 6 million curies of cesium-137 and that most of this inventory was released in the accident. (A curie is a unit of radioactivity equivalent to 37 billion nuclear disintegrations per second.) By way of comparison, the amount of iodine-131 released during the accident at Three Mile Island, Pennsylvania, was 15 curies, and a typical nuclear explosion in the atmosphere (test explosions were permitted until 1963) released 150,000 curies of this element.

Because of the immense heat of the burning graphite, maybe half of the radioactivity released from Chernobyl was injected high into the atmosphere, to a height of 20,000 feet or more, and blown eastward, Knox believes. The other half reached lower altitudes and initially was blown northwest toward Sweden.[7]

The full consequences of the release of radiation from the stricken reactor will not be known for many years. The immediate casualties included 100 people, mostly fire fighters, who were hospitalized with serious radiation injuries. About 30 died from acute radiation sickness.

Some 100,000 Soviet citizens were evacuated because of the accident. Initially, 49,000 people were evacuated from within a 6-mile radius of the reactor, including the town of Pripyat, where the Chernobyl reactor is located. The evacuation did not begin until 4:00 P.M. on 27 April, 38 hours after the accident. Later the evacuation was extended to an 18-mile radius, and to localities even farther afield, as pockets of washed-down radioactivity were discovered.

Kiev, the third-largest city in the Soviet Union, lies 80 miles south of Pripyat, and significant amounts of radiation were soon detected there. Some 100,000 children were sent out of the city to summer camp, the streets were regularly washed down to get rid of contaminated dust, and vegetables were checked for radioactivity.

No evacuations were necessary outside the Soviet Union, but countries as far away as Italy started to monitor vegetables for radioactivity. Many countries refused to accept exports of food from the Soviet Union and Poland.

The longer-term effects of the release have yet to be assessed. Land in the Soviet Union that has been contaminated with cesium, a long-lived radioactive isotope, may have to be held out of production for many years. So far almost no specific information on radioactivity levels has been released by the Soviet Union. Little can reliably be said about the long-term health effects of the radiation, except that thousands of people in the Soviet Union and Eastern Europe are likely to bear the consequences of the accident.

Robert Gale, the American physician who went to Moscow to perform marrow transplants on the Chernobyl radiation victims, has warned that there are "50,000 to 100,000" potential radiation victims in the Soviet Union. Although the quantities of radiation were quite small, and likely to cause only a small increase in the natural rate of cancer, the radioactive cloud spread over an area inhabited by some 100 million people in the Soviet Union, Eastern Europe, and Scandinavia. Among this population, about 5,000 extra deaths from cancer may be expected, according to calculations by Thomas Cochran of the Natural Resources Defense Council and Frank von Hippel of Princeton University.[8]

The disaster at Chernobyl has prompted many changes in the governance of nuclear power, ranging from proposals to strengthen international reporting of reactor accidents to reviews of plant safety. The less well advertised lesson is the long reach of radiation and the enormous social disruption that can be caused by even a single source of radioactive fallout.

5

The Medical Effects
of Nuclear War

The immediate medical effects of a single, small nuclear explosion are well known from Hiroshima and Nagasaki. So too are some of the longer-term effects, such as the increased incidence of certain types of cancer among the survivors. The consequences of multiple nuclear explosions in the United States or the Soviet Union are hard to imagine because of the many secondary effects, such as the disruption of medical care, public order, and communications, that would influence the condition of survivors. Nonetheless, some estimate can be made of how nuclear war would affect public health.

The survivors of a nuclear explosion would suffer from three kinds of immediate injury—wounds from blast, burns caused by the thermal pulse or the ensuing fires and superfires, and radiation sickness. The injuries would, of course, range from mild to severe, but few survivors could be sure of receiving the same quality of medical care as available in peacetime. Medical facilities are certain to be overwhelmed by the numbers of wounded. Burns and radiation illness are particularly demanding of medical resources. In areas where functioning hospitals survived, physicians would probably have to operate by triage. Those with critical wounds and uncertain chances of survival would be left untreated, as would those judged likely to pull through unaided. To save the greatest number of lives with their limited resources, physicians would concentrate time and resources on the moderately wounded.

People who survived the immediate effects of nuclear weapons would face other hazards in the ensuing days and weeks. Many areas for miles downwind of the nuclear detonations would be contaminated with hazardous or lethal amounts of radiation. Radiation being invisible, many people might stay in the danger zones or wander into them unawares, until the contaminated areas had been assessed and publicly delineated.

Food and water might also be contaminated with radioactivity. Until survivors learned which sources were safe, they would be in danger of ingesting radioactive materials and accumulating an internal body dose. If public health measures should fail, epidemics could break out, particularly among refugees living in crowded conditions without sanitation. The psychological stresses on most survivors might well be severe. If the smoke from the nuclear exchange triggered nuclear winter, the darkened skies and ensuing chills would be further tests of stamina. In the longer term, survivors would face a slightly increased risk of cancer.

Physicians can describe the nature of these various medical effects, but the likely number of casualties depends on the scope of the nuclear attack. Though many observers doubt that any nuclear war will be limited, Administration policy rests on the hope that a nuclear war, if started, can be concluded at the lowest possible level of violence. A limited attack targeted mainly on missile silos could kill tens of millions of people, but considerably fewer than would die in an all-out exchange that included cities. A limited attack would leave many intact areas from which rescue attempts might be made to aid survivors; an all-out nuclear exchange would probably impair transport and communications so severely that each city and region would have to fend for itself. Some of the factors that would determine the number of casualties are discussed below in chapter 9. Regardless of the numbers killed, the effect of nuclear explosions on those who survive would be extensive and brutal.

Immediate Casualties

Blast Injury. The shock wave from a nuclear explosion can damage the human body in various ways. The blast, a shell of compressed air traveling rapidly outward from the explosion, compresses the body and impels it forward. People may be slammed into walls or hurled to the ground at high speed. Those out in the open may be wounded by the flying debris or splinters of glass that are generated by the shock wave. Those inside buildings may be crushed as the shock wave makes the buildings collapse.

The primary effect of the blast wave is its sudden compression of the human body. It squeezes in the walls of the chest and stomach so sharply that the inner organs have no time to adjust. The lungs are particularly prone to hemorrhage, and if the damage is severe, bubbles of air reach the veins of the lung and enter the bloodstream. The bubbles get stuck in smaller blood vessels and may block the blood flow through them. In organs such as the brain and heart, for which an uninterrupted supply of oxygen is essential, these blockages can be rapidly fatal. Death can occur in a few minutes.[1]

Movement after blast damage to the heart or lungs is extremely hazardous; persons who try to walk may die from the effort. Another primary effect of blast is damage at the areas where body tissues of different density join one another, such as where cartilage and bone join soft tissue. The blast can rupture eardrums, but rather few such injuries were seen at Hiroshima and Nagasaki. People who survive 24 to 48 hours without treatment usually recover, and their lung hemorrhages are mostly gone after seven to ten days.[2]

Secondary effects of blast come from the impact when flying

bodies meet solid objects, causing fractures of the skull, broken bones, and the other usual injuries. In the winds created by the blast of nuclear explosions, almost any movable object can be transformed into a dangerous missile. The deep wounds these can create ideal conditions for infection. Many victims suffer a multitude of minor cuts and bruises, and may retain fragments of glass or other debris for years.

Burn Injury. The thermal pulse of a nuclear weapon causes direct injury—known as flash burns—to exposed skin and sometimes even to skin beneath clothing. Victims may also suffer flame burns from the fires that follow a nuclear explosion.

Burns are classified as first, second, or third degree, in increasing severity, depending on the depth of skin that is injured. First-degree burns, like sunburn, heal with no scarring. Second-degree burns are more severe, and a scab forms over them. Still, they do not damage the lowest layers of the skin, which regenerates from the remaining cells and heals within two weeks unless complicated by infection. In third-degree burns the full thickness of skin is injured. The skin cannot regenerate normally, and a scar is formed unless new skin is grafted. Third-degree burns covering 25 percent of the body, or second-degree burns covering 30 percent, generally produce shock within a few hours.

For a one-megaton weapon detonated at 10,000 feet on a clear day, probably 18 percent of an average population within ten miles of ground zero would receive second-degree burns to their exposed skin, and 82 percent would receive first-degree burns.[3] Many of these would also suffer and die from flame burns, because of the superfires that would rage out seven and a half miles or more from ground zero.

At Hiroshima and Nagasaki so many of those caught in the flames did not survive that flame burns constituted only 5 percent of the total burn injuries. The rest were flash burns, which accounted for 20 to 30 percent of fatal casualties in the two cities. The large number of flash burns was probably due to the clearness of the day, which offered no obstruction to the bomb light, and to the fact that people were wearing light clothing in the summer heat. The severity of the flash burns ranged from mild reddening to charring of the skin. The first-degree burns healed spontaneously. Moderate second-degree burns healed within four weeks, but more serious burns often became so infected that healing took longer. As Glasstone and Dolan note, "Even under the best conditions, it is difficult to prevent burns from becoming infected, and after the nuclear bombings of Japan the situation was aggravated by inadequate care, poor sanitation, and general lack of proper facilities. Nuclear radiation injury may have been a contributory factor in some cases because of the decrease in resistance of the body to infection."[4]

Many at Hiroshima and Nagasaki suffered from flash blindness, in which useful vision is lost for up to a few minutes and then returns. Bomb light can blind or burn holes in the retina of anyone looking at the detonation. Nonetheless, among the survivors of Hiroshima and Nagasaki, only a single case of retinal injury was reported even though many survivors had facial burns, often with a singeing of the eyebrows or eyelashes. Eye injury from nuclear weapons would be greater at night (though fewer people would then be outside) because the pupil of the eye opens wider when adapted to the dark.[5]

Medical Effects of Radiation

Blast injuries and burns are well-known consequences when cities are bombed, but Japanese authorities after the bombing of Hiroshima and Nagasaki were presented with a wholly new category of illness—radiation sickness.

On the day of the explosion, survivors showed nausea, vomiting, excessive thirst, loss of appetite, general malaise, fever, and diarrhea. In the second stage, which began 10 days later, their hair began to fall out. For most survivors this began on the 14th and 15th days and affected mostly the hair on the head, although sometimes the pubic, facial, and armpit hair was also shed. Eyebrows were quite resistant.

About 5 to 7 days after hair loss began, a fever set in, often followed within 48 hours by small hemorrhages spread throughout the tissues of the body and visible as blotches on the skin known as purpura. The gums turned to red, then to reddish purple. Deaths from the disease peaked on the 10th day, followed by a 10-day lull and a much larger wave of deaths that ran from day 18 to day 45.[6]

Despite these copious symptoms and the many deaths from radiation sickness after the Hiroshima and Nagasaki bombs, the effects of radiation on the human body are still not precisely understood. In particular, there is uncertainty in predicting the clinical effect of a given amount of radiation. Understandably enough, careful clinical observations in Japan did not begin until two weeks after the bombs fell, and by then the victims were already suffering from malnutrition and infections of various kinds. Some symptoms, such as keloid scars, were probably erroneously attributed to radiation.

In an effort that continues to this day, the Japanese survivors have been studied by the U.S.-Japan Joint Commission for the Investigation of the Effects of the Atomic Bomb in Japan, and by its successor organizations, the Atomic Bomb Casualty Commission and the Radiation Effects Research Foundation. By relating the survivors' injuries to their distance from ground zero, researchers have been able to construct a relationship between clinical effect and radiation dose. These data have been supplemented by information from other incidents of human radiation—in laboratory accidents, in patients and physicians using radiation to treat cancer, and in the Marshall Islanders accidentally exposed by the Bravo test of 1954 at Bikini Atoll. There emerges the following picture of the immediate effects of radiation on humans.

At almost all doses there is an initial, latent, and final stage of illness, though in high doses the three phases may be very compressed. In the initial phase a victim experiences nausea, vomiting, headache, dizziness, and a general feeling of illness. Then follows a latent phase with few, if any, symptoms. The individual can often get up and work as usual. In the final phase the initial symptoms return, along with skin hemorrhages, diarrhea, loss of hair, and, with higher doses, seizures and prostration. The final phase ends when the victim either recovers or dies, depending largely on the dose of radiation received.[7]

Radiation dose is measured in various ways, most often in the unit known as the radiation absorbed dose, or rad. Radiation to the whole body affects all organs and tissues but damages them to different degrees. At very high doses, 5,000 rads or above, the central nervous system is affected. Excitability is followed by drowsiness, lethargy, delirium, and frequent seizures, then by convulsions and coma. Death is certain, occurring within the space of a few hours to two days.

At doses between 1,000 and 5,000 rads, the most critically affected organ is the gastrointestinal tract. Like other cells that often divide and double, the cells lining the intestines are particularly vulnerable to radiation. Damage to them, and to the cells of the bone marrow, is quickly lethal. Stomach pain, nausea, loss of appetite, vomiting, and diarrhea become increasingly severe. Within a few days the victim is emaciated and exhausted. Death occurs within 2 to 14 days from circulatory collapse caused by loss of water and electrolytes, starvation, and infection.

At doses of between 200 and 1,000 rads, the critical organ is the bone marrow, where the body's red and white blood cells and platelets are formed. Radiation stops the division of the precursor cells that form these critical elements of the blood. Lack of platelets, which help in clotting the blood, makes the victim prone to hemorrhaging, and the dearth of white blood cells prevents the body's immune defense system from battling infectious agents like viruses and bacteria.

Survival is possible within the lower part of the 200-to-1,000-

rad dose range, especially if the patient can be kept alive with blood transfusions and antibiotics until the bone marrow can recover. Over the range of 200 to 600 rads, the probability of death in untreated adults goes from 1 percent to 99 percent. The figure of 450 rads is often taken as the LD-50/60, the dose that will be lethal to half those exposed to it within 60 days, although, as discussed below, the true figure for wartime conditions may be much lower.

For healthy adults who receive from 100 to 200 rads of whole-body radiation, survival is very probable, and the symptoms of radiation sickness will disappear without event. At doses of less than 100 rads, there are usually no clinical symptoms, although 10 percent of people will suffer loss of appetite, nausea, and vomiting after exposure to as little as 50 or so rads.[8] But those who survive acute radiation sickness may still be vulnerable to the longer-term effects that smaller doses may produce.

Rethinking the Lethal Dose

Since the end of World War II, the U.S. government has made the standard assumption that, without intensive medical treatment, 450 rads absorbed within 48 hours is the dose of radiation that will cause half of those exposed to die within 60 days. This measure, known as the lethal dose and abbreviated LD-50/60, is the basis for calculating radiation casualties in the wake of a nuclear exchange. Since in a large-scale nuclear war so many people will be exposed to radiation, any change in the LD-50/60 will make a considerable difference to the estimated numbers of dead and survivors.

The official figure of 450 rads for the LD-50 has been criticized by those who feel that the real figure, certainly in wartime, could be much lower. Many died from radiation at Hiroshima and Nagasaki, but it has been generally held that these deaths cannot be used to calculate the LD-50; blast and heat could also have contributed, making it impossible to estimate the effect of radiation alone. But Joseph Rotblat, of the University of London, has recently found an ingenious way to make use of the Japanese data.

As part of the continuing study of the medical effects of the two bombs, Japanese scientists have established a list of 1,216 people who were in houses at varying distances from ground zero at the time of the Hiroshima explosion. If the houses protected them from heat and blast, it is possible their deaths were due principally to radiation. Rotblat believes that this is indeed the case, because of the time course of their deaths and because of its variation with distance from ground zero.

Deaths among the victims of the Hiroshima attack were most numerous in the first few days after the explosion and then steadily decreased. But the pattern of death among people in houses is quite different from that of other deaths, mostly among people caught out in the open. It rises to a maximum about 10 to 20 days after the detonation and then decreases. This pattern of deaths over time closely resembles the pattern obtained when laboratory mice are exposed to radiation. Rotblat's thesis is that the deaths of the 1,216 in houses at Hiroshima were nearly all due to radiation exposure, and that therefore an estimate for the LD-50 in humans can be calculated from them.

By noting how the mortality among the group in houses varied with distance from ground zero, Rotblat calculates that the distance at which 50 percent of those exposed died from radiation was 2,927 feet. What was the dose at this distance? Taking into account the various kinds of radiation from the Hiroshima bomb, and the extent to which each is attenuated by Japanese housing materials, he calculates the dose reaching the bone marrow as 154 rads.

The dose at Hiroshima was received instantaneously, which is more traumatic to the body than the same dose delivered over a period of time, as happens in radiation from fallout. Moreover, fatalities from fallout are usually calculated on the basis of radiation to the whole body, only part of which will penetrate to the bone marrow. Taking these two factors into account, Rotblat calculates that the LD-50 is about 220 rads—just under half the usual figure of 450.[9]

There was widespread malnutrition in Hiroshima and Nagasaki before the bombings, manifested in anemia, diarrhea, and a weakened resistance to injury and disease.[10] Since radiation deaths occur in part because the body's immune defense system is impaired, the people of Hiroshima and Nagasaki may have been unusually susceptible to radiation. The populations of the industrialized Northern Hemisphere would be considerably better nourished, and therefore less susceptible to radiation, than the population of Hiroshima prior to the bombing. Nonetheless, malnourishment would probably set in after a nuclear attack, and populations might quickly become more susceptible to radiation. In such circumstances a realistic value for the LD-50 could well be somewhat less than the usual estimate of 450 rads. Even a slight downward revision of the LD-50 significantly increases the likely number of casualties caused by a large-scale nuclear exchange.

Medical Care after Nuclear War

People not immediately killed by the radiation, thermal pulse, or blast of a nuclear weapon would find themselves in a zone of shattered buildings, racked by high winds, flying debris, and intensifying fires. Blocked streets would impede rescue. Probably only those who could escape on foot from the superfire zone would have a chance of survival.

Treatment of the severely wounded would require intravenous fluids, blood transfusions, antibiotics, the cleaning of contaminated wounds, and the setting of bones. If the wounded could rely only on medical resources from the stricken city, with no help from outside, the mortality rate would be high. Nearly all of the severely wounded would die within a few days.

Modern hospital care is one of society's more sophisticated

services, and among those most prone to disruption. The conditions produced by nuclear weapons in the surviving injured—trauma, burns, and radiation sickness—are among the most demanding of medical attention and resources. The numbers of people injured by a single nuclear weapon exploding over a city would overwhelm any nation's medical facilities.

Many hospitals are located in city centers, and would be destroyed in any attack that targeted cities directly. At Hiroshima the bomb killed 90 percent of the city's physicians, 86 percent of dentists, 80 percent of pharmacists, and 93 percent of its nurses.[11] The remaining quality of medical care at Nagasaki was equally rudimentary: "Most of the hospitals, so desperately needed, had been burned or demolished. Of seventy or so doctors in private practice in the city, twenty were dead and about twenty more seriously wounded, leaving hardly thirty to help. Apart from the small-scale Nagasaki Army Hospital in the old city quarter, there were no facilities to serve as bases for emergency care. First-aid stations set up in primary schools were the main places for emergency treatment of people in the vicinities soon after the bombing. A team from the city's medical association quickly assembled at Katsuyama Primary School northeast of the city hall; and by evening of the first day, a first-aid team of thirteen (two doctors, two noncommissioned medical corpsmen, eight nurses, and a noncommissioned bus driver) from Isahaya Naval Hospital arrived at the school. Fear of spreading fires forced them to move to Irabayashi Primary School; but by evening the number of patients exceeded a thousand, and available medical supplies were exhausted."[12]

Left to their own resources, Hiroshima and Nagasaki could offer little effective medical care to their wounded. Help quickly started to arrive from neighboring regions. But after a major nuclear exchange, medical facilities over large regions of each country would probably be devastated; others would be too overwhelmed with local victims to offer help to those farther away. After an attack limited to nuclear forces, help would probably be available from cities that remained untouched, provided that communications had not been disrupted and a civil defense effort had been organized.

A large proportion of the injured will have suffered extensive burns from the thermal pulse or the ensuring fires. These injuries are the most difficult to treat since for proper care they require a specialized environment and more medical supplies and attention than any other category of injury. Burn care is often prolonged; in the burn unit of a military hospital where the average patient was burned over 30 percent of the body, the average length of stay was 61 days and the number of operations was four per patient. Severely burned patients need full care immediately; chances of survival drop significantly with every few hours' delay.

Burn care facilities are scarce even in peacetime. In the entire United States, there are 135 burn units, with a total of 1,346 beds. Intensive care units, needed for those with less severe burns and for many radiation and trauma injuries, would also be in short supply; in the United States there are 62,000 intensive care beds.

People injured in a nuclear explosion would create a particularly heavy demand for blood products. The trauma from blast injuries often requires that a patient have blood transfusions. Burn patients require fluid replacement in massive amounts, particularly in the hours and days immediately following injury. Radiation victims also need large amounts of blood products, particularly of platelets and white blood cells, components that have short shelf lives and must essentially be collected when needed.

All three groups of injured—those suffering from trauma, burns, or radiation—would need large amounts of antibiotics to stave off infection, the most dangerous complication of their conditions.

A single one-megaton bomb detonated high above Detroit (thus creating little or no fallout) would kill 470,000 of the city's

4.3 million citizens and leave 630,000 injured, according to an estimate by Congress's Office of Technology Assessment. Many of the injured would have more than one type of wound. Among the 630,000, there might be expected 440,000 cases of injury from blast, 409,000 burn cases, and 157,000 with moderate to serious radiation sickness. According to Herbert Abrams, proper medical care of the injured would require 42,000 burn beds, 134,000 intensive care beds, 1,280,000 units of whole blood and of red blood cells, and 15,000,000 units of platelets.[13]

National supplies, let alone the state of Michigan's, would be vastly inadequate to meet the demands of casualties from a single weapon. The gross deficiency in hospital supplies would be only a small part of the problem in providing medical care for the wounded. The electromagnetic pulse generated by nuclear weapons would probably have destroyed all unprotected electrical equipment as well as large parts of the telephone system and electric power grid. Within affected regions water

Medical Supply and Demand
after One-Megaton Airburst over Detroit

	Supplies Required	Supplies Available in Michigan State	Supplies Available in United States
Burn beds	42,000	41	1,346
Intensive care beds	134,000	1,900	62,000
Hospital beds	352,000	37,000	1,350,000
Whole blood (units)	1,280,000	1,800	58,000
Red blood cells (units)	1,280,000	6,000	195,000
Platelets (units)	16,000,000	350	12,000

supplies would become critical. Pumps would fail and water mains rupture. Many supplies drawn from surface water would be contaminated with radioactive fallout. Once their own emergency generators had run out of fuel, hospitals in many areas would have no source of power, hence no means of operating the many electrical machines on which modern medicine depends.

Wartime Japan had far fewer medical supplies than would be available even in a nuclear-devastated region at present. Still, the makeshift care available to the survivors of Hiroshima and Nagasaki is similar in principle to that which survivors of a nuclear exchange might face. "Medical care in the early days after the atomic bombings was extremely handicapped by the huge numbers of casualties and severe shortages in both medical personnel and medical supplies. The main problem in the early stage was burns, and application of zinc oxide oil or ointment was about the only treatment. Zinc oxide oil was often not available, so in many cases rapeseed oil, cooking oil, castor oil, and even machine oil were used. For disinfecting wounds and burns, whatever was at hand—iodine, tincture, mercurochrome, rivanol, boric acid solution or ointment—was used. Among traumas, the most difficult to cope with was the removal of countless glass splinters embedded in the skin and muscles. Furthermore, it was especially hard to stop A-bomb wounds from bleeding; the application of compresses moistened with adrenaline proved only slightly effective. Open wounds easily festered, and often gangrene set in. Before long, diarrhea and bloody stools became common complaints. . . . Antibacterial drugs were also inffective in relieving the symptoms. And to make things worse, it was summertime; so flies swarmed on open wounds, laid eggs, and then maggots appeared in wounds to complicate treatment."[14]

Contrary to the situation at Hiroshima and Nagasaki, where there was almost no fallout, medical supplies and personnel could not be brought into many areas because of the lethal levels of radiation that would persist for days or weeks after an attack. Most of the injured would be fortunate to receive even the most rudimentary treatment. The severely injured, and even many of those with moderate wounds, would soon be added to the list of dead.

Public Health after Nuclear War

Those who survived a large-scale nuclear exchange with minor or no injuries would face public health problems of unprecedented severity. The most critical problem in many regions would probably be access to clean, uncontaminated water. The radioactive elements iodine-131 and strontium-90 would pollute many freshwater supplies, making rain and stream water too radioactive for consumption for about a month. Low-level radioactivity, mostly from strontium-90 and cesium-137, would persist for years.

The next most serious problem would be food. In many regions, only canned or stored food would be safe for consumption. Distribution of food from unaffected regions would be difficult unless adequate transport had survived or could be organized.

A third major source of hazard would be the possible breakdown of public health. Maintaining adequate sanitation is often difficult among people living in the hardship and crowding of refugee camps. With many people weakened from radiation, stress, and malnutrition, there could be outbreaks of infection and communicable diseases. Long-vanquished epidemic scourges like cholera, typhoid fever, tuberculosis, and even bubonic plague could once again flourish if the public health barriers against them were to erode.

Epidemics could be particularly serious if the immunological state of the population were depressed. Radiation depresses the immune system, as do burns, stress, malnutrition, and ultraviolet light of the type that might follow a depletion of the ozone layer by nuclear explosions. These various stresses would not all be experienced at the same time. Victims of radiation and burns, if they did not die, would tend to recover from their injuries after a number of weeks. If scenarios of nuclear winter prove correct, the soot clouds will shield the earth from ultraviolet rays for months, even if the ozone layer is destroyed.

Although there is an evident possibility of epidemics after a nuclear war, no fair discussion can ignore the fact that at Hiroshima and Nagasaki, where epidemics were also expected, none occurred. The standard account of the medical effects of the bombings notes, "The absence of major epidemics in Hiroshima and Nagasaki appears surprising in view of the conditions making for a low level of public health. These factors included breaks in the water-distribution system, resulting in possible pollution and increased use of wells; the lack of disinfectants owing to the destruction of manufacturing and shipping facilities by previous bombings; and the swarms of flies, mosquitoes, and other insects attracted by uncollected garbage and excreta. Despite these conditions there was no major outbreak of epidemic diseases following the bombings."[15]

The authors of this account suggest that the absence of epidemics was "probably due to the sudden large exodus of population" from the bombed cities. Nonetheless, modern cities, too, might be evacuated and the survivors dispersed to outlying regions. Epidemics thus seem a likely danger but not inevitable.

The Use of Shelters

Shelters can provide effective protection from radiation; in Nagasaki, ten people in tunnel shelters located less than 330 yards from ground zero are reported to have survived. Ordinary residential houses can reduce radiation by a factor of three; basements, by a factor of 10, and a cellar or tunnel covered by a yard of earth, by a factor of 1,000.

The intense heat within the zone of a fire storm is likely to make survival in shelters impossible. For those in the zone of local fallout who have taken refuge in shelters, a rule of thumb is that if the radiation level is 1,000 rads per hour at one hour after the explosion, it will fall to 100 rads per hour seven hours later, to 10 rads per hour by two days later, and to 1 rad at roughly two weeks after the explosion.[16] In heavily contaminated but survivable areas, it may be necessary to stay in shelters for two weeks without interruption. It would then be safe to emerge for a few hours a day over a period of months.

The health of people surviving in shelters could present problems, particularly in urban shelters holding large numbers of refugees. Those in charge of a shelter would have to distribute available stores of uncontaminated food and water, care for the sick, dispose of wastes, maintain barriers against infection and panic, and manage on their own resources for days until outside help was available.

The Psychology of the Aftermath

The survivors of a nuclear attack would have endured an unprecedented physical disaster, which would probably have struck with little or no warning. Unlike the victims at Hiroshima and Nagasaki, these survivors could not count on receiving help from outside. Because of the intense electromagnetic effects caused by nuclear weapons detonated above the atmosphere, radio, television, and telephone systems might be knocked out over vast areas. Survivors in many regions would be isolated, cut off from news, ignorant of whether others were aware of their plight or planning to help them.

Survivors of conventional disasters like floods or earthquakes go through wild oscillations of mood and belief. As the full extent of the destruction becomes apparent, and help fails to materialize, the first shock is succeeded by a second shock effect of dismay and abandonment. People's feelings tend to veer from one extreme to another, from terror to elation, invulnerability to helplessness, fear of isolation to hope of escape.

Some may rationalize their survival by a feeling of personal invulnerability and feel intense elation from meeting with rela-

tives or friends who were feared lost. But elation is short-lived
and gives way to the "disaster syndrome," in which victims
appear dazed, bewildered, and indecisive. The passive response
may be a protective reaction, cutting people off from news that
would evoke further pain and anxiety. Or maybe people feel
helpless in the face of massive damage and the seeming impossi-
bility of reconstruction. In the bombing raids on London in
World War II, social cohesion and morale broke down quickly
in the worst-affected areas, although censorship ensured that
this was not widely known at the time.

When the immediate danger has passed, some survivors will
begin to cope with consequences. But family bonds are likely to
prove stronger than civic duties because everyday tasks may
seem futile. Gradually, individual reactions become coordinated
into an organized response.[17]

The reactions to conventional disasters offer only a faint guide
to those that might be prompted by a nuclear exchange. The
bombs dropped on Hiroshima and Nagasaki produced scenes of
extraordinary horror, yet these weapons, with explosive power
equivalent to 12.5 and 22.0 kilotons of TNT respectively, were
minute compared with modern nuclear weapons. T. Akizuki, a
doctor working in a Nagasaki hospital when the bomb fell,
describes how survivors streamed in clamoring for water and
medical attention: "Half naked or stark naked, they walked with
strange, slow steps, groaning from deep inside themselves as if
they had travelled from the depths of hell. They looked whitish;
their faces were like masks. I felt as if I were dreaming, watching
pallid ghosts processing slowly in one direction—as in a dream
I had once dreamt in my childhood."

Other important testimony about the attitude among the Japanese survivors comes from Michihiko Hachiya, director of the
Hiroshima Communications Hospital. Dr. Hachiya, severely
wounded in the attack, kept a diary of the aftermath of the
explosion. In a moving and often quoted passage, he reflects on
a day by which he had recovered enough from his wounds to

walk around the city talking to people of their experiences: "I thought of the dead. . . . I thought of stories I had heard the first day. What a weak, fragile thing man is before the forces of destruction. After the *pika* [the nuclear flash] the entire popula-tion had been reduced to a common level of physical and mental weakness. Those who were able walked silently towards the suburbs and the distant hills, their spirit broken, their initiative gone. When asked whence they had come, they pointed to the city and said, 'that way'; and when asked where they were going, pointed away from the city and said, 'this way.' They were so broken and confused that they moved and behaved like automa-tons.

"Their reactions had astonished outsiders who reported with amazement the spectacle of long files of people holding stolidly to a narrow, rough path when close by was a smooth easy road going in the same direction. The outsiders could not grasp the fact that they were witnessing the exodus of a people who walked in the realm of dreams.

"A spiritless people had forsaken a destroyed city; the way and the means were of no importance. Some had followed the railways, some, as if by instinct, had chosen footpaths and paddy fields, whereas others found themselves shuffling along dry river beds. Each to his separate course for no better reason than the presence of another in the lead.

"As the day ended I might as well have been suspended in time, for we had no clocks and no calendars."[18]

The mood of this passage has been echoed in several second-ary accounts. Survivors of a nuclear war, according to Robert Lifton and Kai Erikson, "would remain in a deadened state, either alone or among others like themselves, largely without hope and vaguely aware that everyone and everything that once mattered to them had been destroyed. . . . Virtually no survivors would be able to enact that most fundamental of all human rituals, burying their own dead. The bonds that had linked people in connecting groups would be badly torn, in most cases irreparably, and the behavior of the survivors likely to become muted and accompanied by suspiciousness and extremely primitive forms of thought and action. . . . The question so often asked, 'Would the survivors envy the dead?' may turn out to have a simple answer. No, they would be incapable of such feelings. They would not so much envy as, inwardly and outwardly, resemble the dead."[19]

Yet in the depths of despair and horror, many survivors after a time wish to continue surviving. That at least was the case with Dr. Hachiya. The diary entry quoted above was written on 11 August 1945, five days after the bombing. By 15 August he recorded, "Hiroshima was destroyed, and here we were working our hearts out to sustain life in the ruins."

When the hospital staff assembled that day around the radio and heard the Emperor broadcast that the war had been lost, there were outbursts of protest at his decision to surrender. "The hospital suddenly turned into an uproar, and there was nothing one could do. Many who had been strong advocates of peace and others who had lost their taste for war following the *pika* were now shouting for the war to continue. . . . The one word— surrender—had produced a greater shock than the bombing of our city."

That sentiment, less often quoted, shows a surprising resilience, particularly as attributed to hospital staff who were working among the worst sights of human suffering that the nuclear weapon had caused.

Despair and horror would certainly be powerful feelings among the survivors of a nuclear exchange. Presumably, the urge to live and rebuild would also reassert itself. The eventual point of balance between the contending emotions would doubtless depend on objective circumstances. But these might not be encouraging, especially if the skies were darkened and the earth chilled for days on end, as the hypothesis of nuclear winter predicts.

Fallout and the Food Chain

The immediate radiation from local and global fallout is external to the body. But people may eat, drink, and breathe contaminated particles, which, if they are retained within the body, will give rise to an internal dose. A particularly serious problem in the wake of a large-scale nuclear war would be the contamination of drinking water.

For the first few months after a nuclear explosion, the dust, smoke, and radioactivity might severely pollute surface waters for a few hundred miles downwind. Rainwater might be a deadly poison, if heavily contaminated, and could even deliver hazardous doses to people who got caught in a light downpour. The principal radioactive element would be iodine, which the body concentrates in the thyroid gland. Radioactive iodine has a half-life of 8 days. Also of concern is strontium, metabolized like the chemically similar element calcium. Radioactive strontium accumulates in the bones, where it damages the blood-forming cells in the marrow.

Much radioactivity will become fixed in dust or settle in the sediment on river beds and lakes. Underground water supplies will be unpolluted at first, but may be hard for survivors to tap unless drilling equipment is at hand. Some experts fear that, in time, even the groundwater may become contaminated with radioactivity and may remain so for some tens of years after a nuclear war. Others rate this risk lower because most dangerously radioactive fission products are strongly absorbed by soil, which would to some extent filter them out. "In general, contamination of groundwater would be tolerable, with certain exceptions," concludes Klaus Wetzel of the Academy of Sciences in Leipzig, East Germany.[20]

The main radioactive elements that affect freshwater supplies are strontium-90 and cesium-137. Strontium-90, with a radioactive half-life of 28 years, also finds its way into the human diet through plants, which absorb it from the soil, and through the milk of cows that have grazed contaminated pasture. Cesium-137, with a half-life of 30 years, is metabolized like the chemically similar potassium and becomes distributed throughout the body.

The internal body dose that might be accumulated from these and other isotopes is almost impossible to calculate because so many factors affect it. One estimate is that internal doses are likely to be 20 percent of the external dose caused by local fallout, about the same as the first month's external dose from global fallout, and somewhat greater than the external dose from long-term global fallout.

The Long Reach of Radiation

Radiation, even in small doses, may damage the body in ways that do not become apparent for months or years after the exposure. The effects known from the Hiroshima and Nagasaki bombings include damage to children in the womb, cataracts of the eye, leukemia, and certain other cancers. An increase in the number of children with genetic defects born to exposed parents would be expected but has not so far been seen. Genetic effects could nevertheless come to light in these children's children.

Radiation to fetuses in the womb profoundly influences growth and development. The most striking finding is small head size, produced in fetuses that were exposed during the first 17 weeks of pregnancy. Some of the small-headed children also appear to be of lowered intelligence. The incidence of small head size is high, and proportional to the dose of radiation the mother received. At Hiroshima, 6 percent of the mothers exposed to as little as 9 rads gave birth to small-headed children. When the dose was between 30 and 150 rads, the chances of a small-headed child rose to about 50 percent. At Nagasaki, essentially no small-headed children were born except to women exposed to very high doses—150 rads or more. But in this case the abnormality was almost certain: eight out of nine women had small-headed infants. The difference in this phenomenon between the two cities may depend on the amount and types of radiation produced by the two bombs, which is still a matter of scientific debate.[21]

Cataracts—changes in the normal transparency of the lens of the eye—began to appear about ten months to five years after the Hiroshima and Nagasaki detonations. In nearly all cases the victims had also suffered extensive loss of hair at the time, suggesting they had received a dose of 300 rads or more. Once they had appeared, the cataracts did not grow any worse, and most have been susceptible to treatment.

Radiation and Cancer

Radiation from nuclear weapons does not cause new types of cancer but increases the incidence of those that occur anyway. About three years after the Hiroshima and Nagasaki bombings, the number of cases of leukemia in both cities began to rise, reaching a peak around 1951–52. The incidence of leukemia had fallen back to the normal level in Nagasaki by the early 1970s, but it is still slightly above normal in Hiroshima. As with the small-headed children, the difference may be because the Hiroshima bomb, a gun-type weapon with uranium-235 as the nuclear material, produced radiation different in kind and amount from that of the Nagasaki device, in which plutonium-239 was made critical by implosion. There is a definite relation between the incidence of leukemia and dose. The lowest dose that clearly increases the risk of leukemia was about 40 rads.[22]

A significant increase in cancer of the thyroid gland was noticed among survivors exposed to more than 50 rads. Delayed abnormalities of the thyroid have also been detected among Marshall Islanders whose glands absorbed internal doses of radioactive iodine from the fallout to which they were exposed. One estimate is that each rad or so of exposure induces ten extra cases of thyroid cancer per million adults exposed, but substantially more for children. If proper treatment is available, thyroid cancer is rarely fatal.[23]

Studies of the mortality data between 1950 and 1970 for the people who were in the two cities indicate an increased incidence of other types of cancer, including those of the lung, gastrointestinal tract, and female breast. Among 690 people who were over 50 years old at the time of their exposure to 100 rads or more, 47 cancer deaths occurred in the period 1960–70, some 50 percent more than the 30 cancer deaths that would otherwise have been expected in such a group. The cancer increase was even more pronounced among those who were only children when exposed to the Hiroshima and Nagasaki bombs. Among 820 children who were under ten in August 1945, there should have been less than 1 cancer death during this period (0.75 of a death, according to the statistics), but in fact 6 deaths occurred. The total excess death from radiation-induced cancer among all survivors up until 1978 is estimated to be 3.4 percent; in other words, 3.4 bomb-caused cancers have occurred for every 100 cancer cases that would be expected anyway.

Cancer deaths caused by radiation were a minute part of the toll of the Hiroshima and Nagasaki bombs. But this aspect of nuclear weapons could be much more significant after a large-scale nuclear exchange in which millions of people throughout the world, possibly everyone, would be exposed to measurable doses of radiation from global fallout. Attempts to estimate this burden are fraught with uncertainty but are nonetheless worth making.

Assuming a large, 6,500-megaton war, with 5,000 megatons exploded in surface bursts (giving very high local and short-term global fallout), C. E. Land and Per Oftedal have estimated that the local fallout would increase the normal cancer rate by 17 percent.[24]

The Genetic Legacy of Nuclear War

The genetic effect on human populations is among the most serious possible consequences of a nuclear exchange, but also among the hardest to assess. That radiation can alter genes was first discovered in 1927 by H. J. Muller's classic experiments on fruit flies. Most such alterations, called mutations, are harmful to the organisms possessing them. Exposure of the global human population to the levels of fallout predicted for a large-scale nuclear war might increase the natural rate of mutation, which would affect the genetic constitution of future generations.

Experiments with mice show that genetic damage is proportional to dose although at low levels, if the radiation is administered over a longer period, some genetic repair can take place. Since human reproduction is quite similar to that of mice, humans should be affected by radiation in approximately the same way. A rough estimate is that an acute dose of 50 rads or so to the ovaries or testes would double the natural rate of mutations in a human population.[25] Other estimates of the dose required to cause a doubling of the natural rate range from 16 to 250 rads. What is the evidence from Hiroshima and Nagasaki?

There have been born about 19,000 children one or both of whose parents were irradiated in the bombing. Comparing the radiation the parents probably received with the doses that cause various genetic defects in laboratory mice, Oftedal estimates that about 265 extra children with genetic damage should have been found among the 19,000.[26] In fact, no significant increase in genetic damage has come to light among the children of survivors.

One explanation is that humans are simply much less susceptible to genetic damage than are mice. In fact, the dose to cause a doubling of the mutation rate must be at least five times higher in humans to account for the Japanese data. Another possibility is that cases of genetic damage occurred but were not recorded.

Oftedal notes that, surprisingly, there are no reported cases of Down's syndrome among the children of the exposed. In the wake of their experiences, parents perhaps rejected or killed children born with abnormalities. According to Oftedal, "Under the circumstances, we may suspect in the first post-war decade a stronger than usual early selection against all types of malformation. However, since a major effort was made to register and examine [the appearance as newborns of] all children born to exposed parents, it is very difficult now to see how an effect of the postulated magnitude could have been missed."

Even if no genetic damage is detectable in the survivors' children, it is still possible that some damage may appear in the second generation, the survivors' grandchildren.

A major study of genetic effects among Japanese bomb survivors has been undertaken by William Shull, Masanori Otake, and James V. Neel. If the survivors sustained genetic harm from the radiation, the damage should make itself manifest by increasing four indicators of genetic health: the number of failed pregnancies, the number of children of survivors dying before adulthood, the abnormalities in the children's chromosomes, and the mutations in their blood proteins. But Shull and colleagues have found no significant increase in any of these indicators. In all the children of survivors, just a single probable case of a protein mutation has been detected.[27]

Given the finding of no genetic damage among the children of the exposed at Hiroshima and Nagasaki, there is little credible basis for assessing the extent of possible genetic defects after a large nuclear exchange.

6

Nuclear War
and Climate

Just a decade ago, a committee of experts convened by the National Academy of Sciences concluded that even a massive nuclear exchange would not significantly affect the world's climate. Opinion has now changed sharply. Taking into account previously neglected factors, like the smoke from burning cities, most students of the subject now agree that nuclear war could in principle derange the climate, blotting out the sun and chilling the ground for weeks on end.

An important debate is now in progress to define the likely extent of this effect, often referred to as nuclear winter. Besides its instrinsic importance, the nuclear winter debate is also a critical part of the present reassessment of the effects of nuclear war. That the nuclear winter effect was discovered so recently and so fortuitously indicates what little attention has hitherto been paid by scientific and military organizations to the probable consequences of nuclear war, even though the threat of waging nuclear war is the essence of nuclear deterrence.

In 1974 Fred Ikle, then director of the Arms Control and Disarmament Agency, asked the National Academy of Sciences to assess the probable long-range consequences of a nuclear exchange on the environment. The academy's committee, in its section on climate, reported that nuclear explosions were likely to affect climate in much the same way that volcanoes do—by injecting massive amounts of rock dust into the atmosphere.

Even a nuclear exchange of 10,000 megatons would loft between 10 and 100 million tons of dust—roughly the same amount as was created by the eruption of the volcano at Krakatoa in 1883. After that eruption, there was a global cooling of a few tenths of a degree; that, argued the committee, is about what should be expected after a massive nuclear exchange. "We tentatively conclude that the stratospheric dust injection from a [10,000-megaton] nuclear exchange would be comparable with that from a large volcanic explosion such as that of Krakatoa in 1883 and therefore might have similar climatic impact. At most, a [half a degree centigrade] deviation from the average lasting for a few years might be expected."[1]

Though this conclusion is now regarded as incomplete, the lacuna should be attributed not so much to the academy committee as to the whole community of people who thought about nuclear weapons. The committee and its panels included expert climatologists and representatives of the two nuclear weapons research laboratories at Los Alamos and Livermore. The fact is that as of 1975 no one had considered that, because nuclear weapons make cities burn, the fires might create a lot of soot and the soot might absorb sunlight more effectively than does rock dust.

A preliminary step toward this recognition was taken when the physicist Luis Alvarez and others suggested in 1980 that the extinction of the dinosaurs 65 million years ago might have been caused by an asteroid that collided with the earth and raised a global dust cloud. The dust, they supposed, blocked out the sun and destroyed the plant and animal life on which the dinosaurs depended.

A second stride was made by Paul Crutzen and John Birks. In a commissioned article for the journal *Ambio,* they surmised that a nuclear exchange would set off forest fires over vast areas;

the smoke would linger in the lower atmosphere—the tropo-sphere—and would probably restrict sunlight for long enough that "agricultural production in the Northern Hemisphere would be almost totally eliminated, so that no food would be available for the survivors of the initial effects of the war."[2]

Crutzen and Birks did not state the nuclear winter hypothesis in its current form—that soot from burning cities reaches the stratosphere—and the significance of the smoke contribution from forests is now a matter of debate. But the attention to smoke was important because whereas dust just scatters light, smoke both scatters and absorbs it. Smoke makes the light deposit its heat, thus heating up the atmosphere at the smoke's level to unusual temperatures. Crutzen and Birks also correctly pointed out that urban and industrial fires, which they were unable to assess at the time, "may be enormously important" in affecting the global environment.

These ideas provided the impetus for others to develop the full-fledged hypothesis of nuclear winter, described in 1983 in an important article by Richard P. Turco, Owen B. Toon, Thomas P. Ackerman, James B. Pollack, and Carl Sagan.[3] They considered the rock dust from nuclear surface bursts, the smoke from ignited forest fires, and the soot from burning cities. Using a relatively simple computer model, they argued that even a small nuclear exchange would create enough dust, soot, and smoke to reduce the transparency of the atmosphere signifi-cantly.

For many of the large-scale nuclear exchanges considered, Turco and his colleagues reported, the clouds would spread over the globe within one or two weeks, quickly reducing light levels to just a small percentage of normal. Land temperatures would drop to between 15 and 25 degrees centigrade below freezing and would stay below freezing for about two months. The effect was particularly apt to be triggered by an attack on cities; a 100-megaton attack, in the form of a thousand 100-kiloton bombs dropped on 1,000 cities, would produce almost as severe a freezing as an all-target, 10,000-megaton exchange.

By analogy with the observed behavior of dust storms on the planet Mars, the Turco group suggested that the clouds of dust and smoke from a Northern Hemisphere war between the superpowers might quickly be spread into the Southern Hemisphere, so that the nuclear winter effect would be global. They forecast that the climatic disturbance would last for more than a year before normal conditions were restored. They noted that the "long-term exposure to cold, dark, and radioactivity would pose a serious threat to human survivors and other species."

Critics like Edward Teller accused the authors and other proponents of neglecting processes that would tend to wash the smoke out of the atmosphere. These processes, many of which are difficult for computer models to handle, include the storms that would occur at coastlines where the frozen land meets the still warm oceans; the patchiness of the smoke clouds, which would let some light in, creating turbulence and further washout; the capping clouds that form above hot smoke plumes, and whose water drops capture and clump together the small smoke particles that otherwise would stay aloft the longest. Because of these neglected effects, Teller argued, the nuclear winter hypothesis should be considered "dubious rather than robust." Nevertheless, he conceded that a cooling action from the smoke clouds was indeed a possibility and that even if the degree of cooling was one-tenth of what the Turco group predicted, the decrease "could still lead to widespread falure of harvests and famine."[4]

The next milestone in the understanding of nuclear winter was a second report by the National Academy of Sciences, this time commissioned by the Department of Defense. This report, published in 1985, essentially endorsed and corroborated the basic principle of nuclear winter but warned against making any conclusion about its likely extent for the time being. The academy's committee, chaired by George Carrier, said that it "cannot subscribe with confidence to any specific quantitative conclusions drawn from calculations based on current scientific knowledge."[5]

Nevertheless, the Carrier committee went through the exercise of trying to predict the extent of nuclear winter, partly to show how serious it could be, partly to indicate where the uncertainties are greatest and what needs to be done to reduce them. Following the committee through this exercise illustrates the complexity of the issue.

First, the Carrier committee assumed a nuclear war with an exchange of warheads equivalent to 6,500 megatons of TNT in total yield. Each side would give highest priority to counterforce attacks, against both the opponent's strategic nuclear forces and his command and control facilities. Each side would also launch a countervalue attack, against the part of the opponent's economic base that supports his military activity. Though neither side would target cities in themselves, the countervalue targets would lie in the 1,000 largest urban areas of the two superpower alliances. Warheads would be fused to detonate at ground level for attacks on hardened targets like missile silos, so that 1,500 of the 6,500 megatons would be in the form of surface bursts.

The surface bursts against silos contribute to nuclear winter by pulverizing and vaporizing the rock around their targets. Large particles of rock will soon drop back to earth, but the fine particles, if carried high enough by the fireball, will linger in the stratosphere, scattering and weakening the sunlight. The critical question is how much fine dust will be lofted into the high troposphere and stratosphere.

If the missile warheads are armored, so that they can penetrate the surface of the ground and explode beneath it, the energy of the explosion goes into creating a shock wave, not a fireball. Although lots of dust will be created, the cloud rise will be very modest. Surface bursts both create a lot of dust and carry it high with the buoyant rise of the fireball. But small warheads, with yields less than one megaton, are not very efficient in transporting dust to stratospheric heights.

From observations of atmospheric nuclear tests prior to 1963, guesses can be made about the amount of rock dust created by a surface burst of given yield, about the proportion of fine dust (less than one micron in radius), and about the height attained by the dust cloud. The Carrier committee assumes that the surface bursts in its war scenario will result in 15 million metric tons of submicron dust being lofted into the stratosphere.

The remaining warheads, totaling 5,000 megatons in yield, will be detonated as airbursts. How much forest smoke and urban soot will be created in the fires caused by these weapons? The targeteers will presumably fuse the warheads to explode at a height that maximizes the shock wave over a given area. About half the weapons' energy goes into creating the shock wave, 15 percent into prompt radiation (as opposed to fallout radiation), and 35 percent into heat and light. Depending on the height of the burst, the thermal pulses that carry the heat and light will ignite most wood and plastic products over a certain area. At Hiroshima and Nagasaki, this was in effect the area that received a thermal pulse of ten calories per square centimeter or more. For the larger weapons of modern arsenals, the Carrier committee assumes that fires will break out only in areas that receive at least twice as much heat—20 calories per square centimeter or more—and that the fires will not spread beyond this zone.

The location of the missile silos and other counterforce and countervalue targets leads the committee to believe that 250,000 square kilometers of forest would fall within the zones heated to 20 calories per square centimeter. Such an area would contain 5,000 million metric tons of wood, leaves, litter, and compost. In natural wildfires about a quarter of this forest fuel is burned, but say only 20 percent—1,000 million tons—is consumed in the nuclear exchange, perhaps because the tinder is wet or because the bomb light is obscured by dust. Observation of natural forest fires suggests that 3 percent of the fuel is turned into smoke, so the forest fires set by the nuclear exchange would generate 30 million tons of smoke.

How much from cities? In the committee's war scenario, 1,500 megatons is detonated over urban areas. If 500 megatons worth is canceled out in the overlap between bombs, and if the average fire zone (the area receiving 20 calories or more per square centimeter) is 250 square kilometers per megaton, then 250,000 square kilometers of cities and suburbs will be consumed.

For the past 50 years the industrial world's cities have been accumulating highly combustible materials—timber, oil, coal, asphalt, plastics, solvents, fibers, and rubber. Probably 75 percent of the material is wood, and another 10 percent plastics, resins, and rubber. The overall combustible load can vary widely, from a residential area (up to 5 grams of fuel per square centimeter) to an office and commercial zone (up to 80 grams per square centimeter). The committee assumes that the average fuel load in an urban area is 4 grams per square centimeter, that only three-quarters of it burns (even though there was almost total consumption in the fire zones of Hiroshima and Nagasaki), and that 4 percent of the burned fuel is turned into fine sooty smoke particles, half of which are washed down by rain. Multiplying these factors together gives 150 million metric tons of fine soot.

The proportion of soot rained out strongly influences the extent of climatic change. Some of the particles will be immediately rained out when the low-level moisture in the air, entrained to higher levels in the rising plume, condenses into droplets and falls as rain. Others will be clumped together in water droplets. When the water evaporates, the single large particle created from several small ones is far less effective in blocking light. Many of the particles are oily to start with and repel water; as they age, however, the oil is oxidized and the particles are more likely to be washed down in rain. It is because of such processes that the committee in its calculation assumes that half the urban smoke will be removed from the fire plumes during the plumes' initial rise.

Thus the committee's war scenario creates 30 million tons of smoke from forest fires and 150 million tons of smoke from urban fires. Some of this smoke could reach the tropopause, the boundary between the troposphere and the stratosphere. The fierce fires raging in burning cities could well generate enough heat to propel smoke to considerable heights. Crosswinds and nighttime cooling would reduce the height attained by the smoke plume; rapid burning and high local humidity would increase it. Forest fires, on the other hand, are more likely to stay in the lower part of the troposphere.

Fire plumes rising from burning cities up to the middle troposphere will be swept along by westerly winds traveling at some 70 kilometers an hour. If the fires last for several hours, their plumes will be spread several hundred kilometers downwind. With 1,000 urban fires burning, under the committee's war scenario, substantial parts of North America, the North Atlantic, Europe, and the Soviet Union will soon be covered with smoke. Smoke-free patches will probably disappear after two days and the full North Atlantic be covered in three. The rock dust in the stratosphere will also spread widely, but not so fast.

Given the predicted optical properties of the smoke, and dust, visibility at ground level would be reduced to nothing for several days after the exchange, at least under the densest clouds of smoke, and plants would have too little light to carry on photosynthesis.

Computer Predictions of Postnuclear Weather

After determination of the expected amount of rock dust, and smoke, the next step is to enter these quantities into the computer-run models used to predict atmospheric processes. A model, in the physicist's sense of the term, is a set of mathematical equations that describes a physical process, in this case the behavior of the atmosphere. In many models, a large number of equations have to be solved repeatedly, and the models tend to become very greedy of computer time and capacity. Their advantage is that they provide a rough simulation of the atmosphere —a "model" of how it behaves—and hence a basis for simulating experiments with it, like injecting tons of smoke into the atmosphere.

The simplest models treat the atmosphere as if it had just one dimension—up and down. These one-dimensional models don't require a lot of computing time, but they necessarily give only rough approximations of the three-dimensional atmosphere they attempt to simulate. The Turco group used a one-dimensional model in its initial prediction of the nuclear winter effect. With the most powerful available computers, it is possible to move to three-dimensional models of the atmosphere, which render more sophisticated and fine-grained predictions.

These general circulation models, as they are known, divide the global atmosphere into grid points, at each of which the temperature, pressure, windspeed, moisture content, and cloudiness are represented. The spacing of the grid points is as close as the computer's memory and storage capacity can handle, but at present even for the most powerful machines grid points have to be spaced several hundred kilometers apart horizontally and at a number of different heights in the troposphere and stratosphere.

Given initial values for quantities representing the global weather, the computer model recalculates the values at each grid point as, in the course of time, they interact with one another through processes like wind and heat flow. By matching these simulations of global weather against observation, and correcting them where necessary, designers have adapted several of these models to provide realistic simulations of the normal climate. But a model that simulates the normal climate may not necessarily do so well with a highly abnormal climate, like that caused by the injections of large quantities of dust and soot.

Also, in this case there no observations against which to calibrate and correct the models' simulations. Nonetheless, the predictions of the postnuclear climate are worth something, even if a greater range of uncertainty must be imputed to them.

The Carrier committee's initial assumptions about smoke and dust were fed into various available computer models. With the same one-dimensional model that the Turco group used, these assumptions produce a clear nuclear winter effect, although one somewhat less severe—the greatest temperature drop at surface level being 21 degrees, compared with a drop of 37 degrees produced by the Turco group's smaller, 5,000-megaton war.

The one-dimensional model, as the Turco group noted, is unable to take into account the role of the oceans—which stay at constant temperature because of their vast heat content—in counteracting the chilling of the land. By assuming that the soot clouds are uniformly spread, the model also exaggerates their insulating effect, since soot clouds of varying thickness would block light less efficiently. Ordinary water clouds, also ignored, are another moderating influence on nuclear winter. General circulation models can correct for all these omissions.

At the National Center for Atmospheric Research in Boulder, Colorado, a general circulation model primed with the Carrier committee's assumptions predicted an average drop in the continental surface temperature of 26 degrees centigrade after a summer war and a 17-degree drop for a war in spring. These are somewhat less extreme than the initial forecast of nuclear winter but give little ground for comfort; subfreezing temperatures would have developed over much of North America and Eurasia by the tenth day after a nuclear exchange.

The Status of Nuclear Winter

The inferences the Carrier committee draws from its nuclear winter study are important because they represent the most sophisticated available understanding of the phenomenon. Nu-

clear winter may one day emerge in black and white; for the time
being, the portrait is mostly gray, but with a clear shape looming
in the fog. A major nuclear exchange, the committee concludes,
"could result in dramatic perturbations of the atmosphere lasting over a period of at least a few weeks." There are still many
uncertainties, but unless some of them have been badly mis-
judged, or some important mitigating factor has been overlooked, "there is a clear possibility that great portions of the
land areas of the northern temperate zone (and, perhaps, a larger
segment of the planet) could be severely affected." That might
mean, in the committee's view, "major temperature reductions"
lasting for weeks, followed by subnormal temperatures for
months thereafter, with possibly harsh consequences for survivors and the environment.

"A more definitive statement," the Carrier committee states,
"can be made only when many of the uncertainties have been
narrowed. . . ."

The Range of Uncertainty

The range of these uncertainties is still very considerable. There
will never be certainty on the size or targets of a nuclear exchange, but the Carrier committee may have chosen an unrealis-
tically large nuclear war as the basis for its scenario. Albert
Wohlstetter points out that the committee made little allowance
for the fact that a certain proportion of each side's missiles
would fail to work. More significantly, the purpose of most
nuclear weapons is to destroy other nuclear weapons. Many
would surely succeed in that task. But the Carrier committee
assumes that 25,000 nuclear warheads—half of the combined
arsenal of the United States and Soviet Union—would be detonated in an exchange. This requires each superpower to attack
the other's missiles in their silos, but in such a way as not to
interfere at all in the opponent's counterattack. The example,
Wohlstetter claims, "illustrates a characteristic of these odd

scenarios: attacks which are nominally directed at military targets seem to do very little direct harm to their military targets, but do manage a large contribution to global disaster."[6]

As to the production of smoke and soot, George Carrier notes a chain of four major uncertainties. Reasonable estimates for the total quantity of combustible materials in cities differ by a factor of 2. The fraction that might burn is also uncertain by a factor of 2. Estimates of the amount actually converted to smoke lie between 2 percent and 6 percent—an uncertainty factor of 3. The extent of the capture and clumping together of smoke particles by water droplets that condense in the smoke plume is also uncertain by a factor of 3. Multiplying these four factors together gives an uncertainty range of 36; in other words, the smallest reasonable estimate for smoke production could be 36 times less than the largest.

Roughly corresponding to this range is the Carrier committee's estimate that its chosen nuclear exchange might create as little as 20 million metric tons of fine smoke or as much as 650 million tons. The value it chose for working purposes was 180 million tons.

A third type of uncertainty concerns the computer-run, mathematical models of the atmosphere. Atmospheric scientists, Carrier observes, have succeeded with these models "in very large measure because [they] have been able to make observations of what happens to the real atmosphere, compare it with what these models tell us, ask why they are different, . . . and improve those big models." But there's no opportunity to go through the same process of feedback and evolution when the models are applied to a conjectural, soot-laden atmosphere.

What specific climatic changes should be assumed by those trying to assess the medical and environmental consequences of nuclear winter? Carrier asserts, "The answer, for all time to come that I can anticipate, is going to be a whole range of possibilities."[7] Nuclear winter, in other words, could be very mild, or it could be very severe, and neither extreme can yet be ruled out. Even a mild chilling, however, could have devastating effects on agriculture.

Interim Forecasts for Nuclear Winter

Since the Carrier committee's report, studies of the nuclear winter hypothesis have continued. A computer simulation devised by Robert Malone and colleagues at the Los Alamos National Laboratory affords a sophisticated insight into the phenomenon.[8]

The Los Alamos simulation is an adaption of the general circulation model of the atmosphere developed by the National Center for Atmospheric Research. Unlike previous models, it takes into account the fact that the clouds of smoke released in a nuclear exchange do not merely attenuate the sun's heat but also absorb it. As the smoke clouds gain heat, they expand, gain buoyancy, and rise. Even if fires inject the smoke quite low into the troposphere, the model indicates, the sun's heating will soon invest them with the buoyancy to rise into the stratosphere.

By the twentieth day after a nuclear exchange, the model predicts, some of the smoke will have reached as high as 25 kilometers, far into the stratosphere, and some will have crossed the equator into the Southern Hemisphere.

The ascent of the smoke causes a major change in the structure of the atmosphere. The tropopause—the region that marks the ceiling of the weather layer of the atmosphere—is depressed from its usual height of about ten kilometers to under five. This is a serious consequence because only the smoke left within five kilometers of the ground can be washed down and quickly removed.

In the stable stratosphere, above the reach of weather, the smoke could linger for months, even years, since its slow sedimentation under gravity is the only force to bring it down. The time it would take a micron-sized smoke particle to fall from ten kilometers, where the bulk of the smoke is lofted, down to the depressed tropopause at five kilometers, is around six months. The Malone group simulated only 40 days of the global atmosphere, but that was enough to indicate that the smoke, at least for a July war, would disappear very slowly.

The Malone group assumed that 170 million metric tons of fine smoke (close to the academy committee's estimate of 180 million tons) would be created by a nuclear exchange and evenly injected into the atmosphere at all levels from ground to nine kilometers. Given this starting point for a July war, their computer model predicts that a veil of smoke quickly enshrouds the whole Northern Hemisphere and the south down to ten degrees latitude below the equator. At day 20 after the war, the thickness of the cloud over the United States and Europe is still enough to reduce sunlight to between 25 and 50 percent of its normal value, depending on latitude.

By a week after a July nuclear exchange the smoke veil, according to Malone's model, has cooled most of the interior United States and Soviet Union by 15 degrees or more. Reductions of 5 to 15 degrees are still experienced by the sixth week.

Conditions would be considerably less severe for a January war. Since the sun shines less strongly on the Northern Hemisphere, much more smoke stays in the troposphere long enough to be rained down. Injection of 170 million tons of smoke would cause a cooling of surface air temperatures by less than 15 degrees below normal during the first two weeks. According to Malone, "The smoke is removed more efficiently than in July, and after three weeks the temperature reductions are superimposed upon and finally overridden by fluctuations reminiscent of wintertime storms."[9]

Another computer test of the nuclear winter hypothesis has recently been carried out by Starley Thompson and Stephen Schneider at the National Center for Atmospheric Research. Injecting the 180 million tons of smoke, as prescribed by the National Academy of Science scenario, they calculate that a nuclear exchange would cause an average temperature reduction of more than ten degrees throughout the temperate latitudes of the Northern Hemisphere. This overall average, however, includes intermittent freezing over "some large areas in the interiors of the North American and Eurasian continents, particularly in Canada and Siberia." Such temperature drops, even if they lasted for only a few hours, could destroy crops like wheat and rice.

Estimates by George Bing of the Lawrence Livermore National Laboratory suggest that cities contain considerably less combustible material than was previously supposed. If so, the likely quantity of smoke produced in a nuclear war could be much less than 180 million tons, maybe 60 million or even 20 million tons. Feeding these two lesser estimates into their computer, Thompson and Schneider find that the case of 60 million tons is essentially similar to that of 180 million; it, too, produces intermittent freezing of the continental interiors. The 20-million-ton case involves a smaller temperature drop and a somewhat quicker reversion to normal.[10]

Conclusion of the Computer Models

What are the computer models able to state about the nuclear winter effect up to now? No substantial objection yet raised "has lessened the probability that a major nuclear exchange would cause severe environmental effects although some of the effects would probably be less extreme than was sometimes suggested in discussion of the early results." That is the conclusion of a committee of the International Council of Scientific Unions, in a review of the results of climatic modeling. The committee noted that the cooling effects predicted by current computer models "are no greater, and indeed may be less, than the cooling which occurs every winter." But if a 15-degree temperature drop occurred suddenly, in the middle of a growing season, "its biological consequences would far exceed those usually associated with winter, because the normal onset of winter is gradual, anticipated, and prepared for by humans, animals and plants alike."[11]

The present computer models are far from being able to give the final picture of nuclear winter. Because their grid points are several hundred kilometers apart, they cannot "see" any weather processes that occur on a finer scale and that can change the larger picture. For these and other reasons, the models produce only sketches of what might be, not a detailed portrait, and the sketches could well prove incorrect even in major features.

7

The Havoc Factor
and the Ozone Shield

Nuclear weapons create complex changes in the physical environment. Some of these effects have been inferred or discovered; others, no doubt, remain undetected or are kept as military secrets. Initial radiation, thermal pulse, blast, fire storms, fallout, and climatic change have already been discussed. Two further important effects warrant description. One is the electromagnetic pulse created at the instant of a nuclear explosion. The other is the disruption of the earth's protective ozone layer by the nitrogen oxides generated in a large-scale nuclear exchange.

The Havoc of EMP

Nuclear explosions create a brief, intense pulse of electromagnetic energy that can wreak havoc with electrical systems over a considerable area. For a bomb detonated near ground level, the pulse's range is only 8 miles or so from ground zero, roughly equivalent to the mechanical damage from the blast wave. For an airburst at a height of 50 miles, the affected area on the ground would be a circle 1,200 miles in diameter. But when a weapon is exploded high above the atmosphere the electromagnetic pulse, or EMP, may derange telephone networks and power grids over several thousands of miles.

"For an explosion at 200 miles above the center of the (conterminous) United States, almost the whole country, as well as parts of Canada and Mexico, could be affected by the EMP," state Glasstone and Dolan.[1] At worst, that could mean that almost everything electrical would cease to function. The communications network would be disrupted. Telephones would not work. The power grid would be knocked out from coast to coast. Devices plugged into the electrical system would be damaged. Televisions would go dark. Computers, in particular, would be liable to destruction or the alteration of data. Radio and television transmitting stations would be knocked out.

The effect of the EMP on military systems might not be so grave because of efforts to protect, or "harden," them against the EMP. Nonetheless, almost all military communications might be put at risk. The ability of the national command and control system to launch weapons, or withhold the launch of weapons, might be impaired. The computer memories of missiles might be affected by EMP and their navigational accuracy degraded.

If nuclear war were not chaos already, EMP would make it so. Like most aftereffects of nuclear weapons, EMP came as a surprise. Although some aspects of EMP were understood before the banning of nuclear tests in the atmosphere, the size of the EMP effect was "not correctly predicted until afterwards."[2] Strong EMP effects were first noticed from a high altitude test, named Starfish Prime, in June 1962. Starfish Prime, a 1.4-megaton nuclear weapon detonated 248 miles above Johnson Island in the Pacific, caused 30 strings of streetlights to fail on the Hawaiian island of Oahu, 800 miles away. Some further data on EMP were gathered in three following tests but, because of the size of the effect was underestimated, the instruments did not record the effect fully. Atmospheric tests were banned in 1963, putting an end to direct exploration of EMP.

EMP was understood so tardily because most American nuclear tests took place in the Pacific, where there are few electrical systems to be damaged. Soviet atmospheric tests were conducted over land, however, and presumably Soviet scientists noticed EMP much earlier and studied it more intensively before the ban on atmospheric tests.

EMP is caused by the gamma rays that burst from a nuclear weapon at the moment of detonation. If the weapon is in the atmosphere, the gamma rays will strike air molecules, knocking free electrons in a process known to physicists as the Compton effect. The Compton electrons, carrying a negative charge, travel outward in all directions, leaving behind a slower-moving shell of molecules that now carry positive charges. This separation of charges takes place at the surface of a sphere around the weapon. If the sphere were perfectly spherical, nothing would happen. In practice, and especially for detonations at or near the earth's surface, the sphere may be squashed at the bottom, and in this case the charge separation causes a powerful net vertical flow of current. As the current flows, a short, intense pulse of electromagnetic energy is emitted at right angles or sideways to it.

For explosions at very high altitudes, EMP is generated differently. The gamma rays from the nuclear chain reaction keep traveling until they meet air molecules at the top of the earth's atmosphere. In a vast pancake-shaped area beneath the bomb, Compton electrons are knocked out and are compelled by the earth's magnetic field to travel in a spiral motion around its lines of force. The spiraling electrons act like a radio transmitter, beaming out a powerful pulse that spans a wide range of frequencies. The electromagnetic pulse thus generated shoots down toward earth from all points of the pancake.

The pulse is somewhat like a radio wave of extreme intensity and brevity. It rises to its peak level of intensity in about 10 to 100 billionths of a second after the explosion, and is almost over in a millionth of a second. But during that almost infinitesimal interval, it reaches an intensity of up to 50,000 volts per meter and generates powerful currents that can damage or destroy electronic components.

The pulse is collected by metallic and other conductors, just as radio waves are picked up by antennas. Good collectors of EMP energy include long runs of cable, large antennas, guy wires, overhead power and telephone lines, long runs of electrical wiring in buildings, girders and reinforcing bars, railroad tracks, and aircraft bodies. The energy of the pulse may then become converted to strong currents and high voltages, which may either damage the equipment or interfere with its function, especially if it uses currents or voltages to represent information.

The types of equipment that may be affected include commercial systems of electric power generation and distribution, telecommunications (radio, television, telephone, and telegraph), and computers. Semiconductor devices like computer chips are particularly susceptible to EMP.

Fiber optics, with their vast capacity for carrying information, may eventually replace the land lines used in the civilian and military telephone systems. But that will not greatly reduce the systems' vulnerability to EMP, because the fibers must still pass through amplifiers and switching centers that are too expensive to shield. The Bell System is not attempting to make its new fiber links invulnerable to EMP.[3]

EMP is unlikely to incapacitate all unprotected communications systems, power grids, and electronic equipment. Nonetheless, "a small number of failures distributed through a large and complex system can disrupt the entire system, or degrade its stability and performance. In this regard, power and communications networks are particularly susceptible."[4]

Equipment can be protected against EMP, but usually only at great expense or inconvenience. Unplugging a device from the electric power main supply will decrease the amount of EMP energy it collects, but this remedy, as Glasstone and Dolan note, "is not always feasible because it would deny use of the equipment." Another of their recommendations, universally ignored at least in the civilian sector, is to design equipment with old-fashioned vacuum tubes instead of the more vulnerable transistors. Many good EMP collectors, such as television antenna masts, are also prone to being struck by lightning and so are equipped with lightning protectors. But the surge of EMP energy comes and goes so quickly—in a few billionths of a second, far faster than lightning—that ordinary lightning protectors cannot respond quickly enough to shunt the pulse aside.

There are several methods of "hardening" equipment against EMP. One is to enclose the whole system in a metal box. But EMP can still leak in through any pipes or wires that enter the box, unless care is taken to install suitable protective devices at the entry points. Another approach is to box just the vulnerable subsystems and to make all signal-carrying connections with optical fibers, which, unlike copper wire, do not collect EMP energy. A third method is "tailored hardening," in which protection is given to just the most vulnerable components, as determined by testing the whole device with an EMP simulator.

How well all these methods work is open to doubt. "Whatever method is used, the uncertainty of the result should be clearly emphasized to decision makers lest oversimplification result," notes a committee of the National Academy of Sciences.[5] EMP protection is in any case so expensive that even vital pieces of strategic military equipment are still vulnerable. Minuteman missile silos have been hardened since 1979, but full protection shielding for nuclear command posts and strategic communications has not been attempted because it could cost billions of dollars. Also these facilities would be vulnerable to nuclear blast, which lessens the incentive to proof them against EMP. Of the airborne command posts used by the President and the Strategic Air Command, only one is considered reliably EMP-proof, and that is a Boeing 747 built from scratch at five times the cost of a commercial plane.[6]

The surveillance and communication satellites needed to conduct a nuclear war are also highly vulnerable to EMP. Gamma rays from a nuclear explosion above the atmosphere can damage satellites thousands of miles away by knocking electrons out of their metal skins. The electrons escape into space, leaving positively charged atoms in the metal. This causes "system generated EMP," or SGEMP, a strong positive flow of current over the surface of the satellite. The Defense Nuclear Agency believes flows of up to 100 amps per square meter would harm unprotected satellites. But a high-yield nuclear weapon detonated 60 miles above the earth could generate SGEMP of 350 to 700 amps per square meter in satellites in geosynchronous orbit.[7]

American strategic doctrine calls for the ability to fight a protracted nuclear war should deterrence fail. Foremost among the problems with this concept is the vulnerability of the command and control system, particularly its communications and satellites, to the chaos wrought by EMP.

The Threat to the Ozone Shield

Ozone is a gas whose presence in the stratosphere protects life on earth from ultraviolet light from the sun. Ozone strongly absorbs the portion of the ultraviolet spectrum that is most damaging to living things. The biologically active ultraviolet light, also known as UV-B, is harmful because it is absorbed by the DNA and protein molecules of living cells.

Ozone is produced when an oxygen molecule absorbs ultraviolet light and splits into two oxygen atoms. Each atom may then combine with an oxygen molecule to form the three-atom molecule known as ozone.

At ground level, ozone contributes to smog and damages plants. High in the stratosphere, it efficiently screens out the ultraviolet rays in the sun's light. These are so harmful to living things that, without the ozone shield, the only living things on earth might be the inhabitants of the oceans.

This vital shield is a fragile structure. The ozone molecules in the rarefied stratosphere are so few that if all were somehow collected and brought down to earth they would form a skin round the globe only three millimeters thick. The tenuousness of the shield makes it vulnerable to chemical changes in the stratosphere. Concern about the shield has played an important and continuing role in discussion about the environmental impact of nuclear war.

It was argued in the early 1970s that the oxides of nitrogen exhausted from the high-flying Concorde and the proposed American supersonic transport might seriously degrade the ozone layer. In 1973 came the first suggestion, by H. M. Foley and M. A. Ruderman, that nuclear explosions would also inject nitrogen oxides into the stratosphere and catalyze the breakdown of the ozone layer. By one estimate, the 300 megatons exploded in Soviet and American atmospheric tests of 1961 and 1962 should have caused a 4 percent decrease in ozone abundance. No clear decrease could be detected, however, in part because the ozone records of the period are too few, and in part because large natural fluctuations in ozone concentrations make it hard to identify small changes.

In 1974 a Canadian scientist, John Hampson, contended that a large nuclear exchange between the superpowers might wipe out the ozone layer. This would be the ultimate doomsday machine, in his view, because both perpetrator and victim of a nuclear attack would perish, and no one on earth would escape the devastation of nuclear war. Hampson's arguments resemble those raised about nuclear winter, but evinced less concern at the time. Later that year Fred Ikle, then director of the U.S. Arms Control and Disarmament Agency, emphasized in several speeches the possible threat that would be posed to life on earth by nuclear war and destruction of the ozone shield. The Department of Defense conceded that perhaps half or more of the ozone layer would be destroyed but stated that the Soviet Union would be more to blame because of the larger yield of its warheads. Supposing that the ozone threat might be a useful bargaining tool in arms control negotiations, Ikle asked the National Acad-

emy of Sciences in April 1974 to assess the long-term environmental consequences of nuclear war.[8]

There are parallels between the ozone threat and nuclear
winter in that both effects are generally accepted to be well
founded in principle but their likely extent remains uncertain.
Ozone is formed from and broken down into oxygen by a complex set of chemical reactions. It is now generally agreed that the
concentration of ozone in the stratosphere is set primarily by its
rate of breakdown and that this is principally determined by
nitrogen oxides emitted from natural sources.[9] Each molecule of
nitric oxide can catalyze the destruction of a trillion or so ozone
molecules before being destroyed itself.

Nuclear weapons create copious amounts of nitric oxide by
heating the nitrogen and oxygen of the air to very high temperatures. This occurs both in the fireball and in the blast wave that
rushes out from it, compressing and heating the air in its path.
It is generally assumed that a certain quantity of nitric oxide is
created per megaton, although this figure "is based wholly on
theoretical considerations and . . . there has not yet been any
attempt at experimental verification of the amounts produced."[10] Nuclear weapons also generate nitrogen dioxide
through the combustion of forests and cities.

If enough nitrogen oxides reach the stratosphere, the ozone
layer will be seriously attenuated. Estimates of the size of the
effect have varied widely, in part because of the changing yields
of strategic nuclear weapons. Weapons with a yield equivalent
to 1 megaton of TNT or more create clouds that can reach into
the stratosphere before they stabilize, and inject large amounts
of nitrogen oxides. Smaller weapons stabilize below the stratosphere, and their nitric oxide is unlikely to threaten the stratospheric ozone. In the study commissioned by Ikle, the National
Academy of Sciences considered a massive, 10,000-megaton
nuclear exchange, with warheads ranging from 1 to 20 megatons
in yield. Its committee estimated that 30 to 70 percent of the

ozone might be destroyed within a few months after the exchange.[11]

Ten years later, in a study of the nuclear winter effect, a different academy committee assumed a 6,500-megaton nuclear exchange, with most warheads of less than one megaton. On this basis, the academy computed that the maximum ozone reduction would be only 17 percent, reached one year after the war's outbreak.[12] Given the general trend toward warheads of smaller yields, the ozone problem might look as if it were going to go away.

This may not be the case. The computer simulations of nuclear winter conducted by Malone and colleagues (see chapter 6) indicate that clouds of soot from burning cities will be heated by the sun and rise into the stratosphere. The soot would probably inhibit the formation of ozone by absorbing some of the ultraviolet light that otherwise would split oxygen molecules into the oxygen atoms that make ozone. Also, by absorbing the sun's heat, the smoke clouds would heat up the stratosphere and enhance the chemical reactions by which nitrogen oxides destroy ozone.[13]

Even if the soot severely damaged the ozone layer in the stratosphere, it would itself absorb the ultraviolet light and prevent it from reaching the earth. But if the soot then settled out of the stratosphere faster than the ozone could regenerate, as is likely, the earth would then be bathed in perilous amounts of ultraviolet radiation. No quantitative assessments of the soot /ozone problem have yet been prepared, but, as the International Council of Scientific Unions notes, "larger, longer lasting and more widespread reductions in stratospheric ozone would now seem to be a possibility."[14]

If so, one of the oldest environmental problems of nuclear war has become its newest.

8

Agriculture and
Environment after War

Would a nuclear war drive humans back to the Stone Age or even to the brink of extinction? With the discovery of the nuclear winter effect, some have seriously suggested such outcomes. So many hardships, they say, will crowd in on the survivors of an exchange that in combination they seem almost overwhelming. The resilience of economic systems and their ability to surmount shortages is generally underestimated. But the natural and maybe the social base on which economies are supported will suffer severe damage in a nuclear exchange. Certain exchanges, especially those that cause major climatic disturbances, could well stretch to breaking point the capacity of natural systems to adapt. Even without climatic change, a whole growing season in North America could be disrupted, with severe consequences for people around the world who depend on American and Canadian grain. The billions of people who survive the immediate aftermath of a nuclear war may for years face the older threat of starvation.

"It is reasonable to assume that mankind in combatant and noncombatant nations would recover from a nuclear war much as it recovered from other major disasters. . . . The most productive land would probably be occupied and tilled within a short time after a nuclear exchange." So declared a panel of agricultural scientists in 1975, in assessing the long-term effects of a 10,000-megaton nuclear war.[1] If the comparison of a 10,000-megaton nuclear war with "other major disasters" now seems inapposite, the error underlines the pitfalls of prediction. Prediction, as is often remarked, is very difficult, particularly with regard to the future. The computer models that simulate the global circulation are a powerful and soundly based tool for forecasting the effect of nuclear war on climate. Yet even they are fraught with uncertainties and limitations. There are no such computer models to predict the reaction of ecological systems to the stress of nuclear war.

The lack of a reliable guide, however, is no excuse for shirking the journey. All the consequences of nuclear war need to be assessed as well as possible, and the long-term effect on the environment is as important as any. Indeed, it is the essence of the new appraisal of nuclear war. Reflecting the consensus view of the time, the report produced by the National Academy of Sciences in 1975 concluded that the environment would survive the two major stresses of nuclear war then envisioned—global radioactive fallout and an increase in ultraviolet light occasioned by a reduction of the layer of ozone gas in the stratosphere.

"Reasoning from available information and understanding," stated Philip Handler, then president of the academy, "it is concluded that, a decade or so after the event, in areas distant from the detonations, surviving humans and ecosystems would be subject to relatively minimal stress attributable to the exchange." Nonetheless, Handler left room for an event that could overturn this optimistic forecast. An unforeseen change in the composition and dynamics of the atmosphere might, "unpredictably, trigger a much larger process and thereby initiate a major change in climate. Hence, one may not exclude the possibility of an unfavorable climate change considerably greater than that explicitly contemplated in this report."[2]

In smoke and dust, the agents of major climatic change have

suddenly appeared, and the threat to natural systems now looks entirely different. Ultraviolet light or radiation may be just another stress to plants, like drought or blight, but a significant reduction of sunlight poses a direct threat to their survival, particularly when combined with prolonged drops in temperature. Climatic change, if severe enough, could disrupt agriculture, tropical forests, and marine life. Crops in northern latitudes would have to be shifted southward or maybe could not be grown at all. Tropical forests, never exposed to very low temperatures, could be devastated by a freeze or prolonged chill. Phytoplankton, the small marine plants that occupy the surface of the oceans, might perish from prolonged lack of light, and their extinction would imperil the long ocean food chains that depend on them.

Postwar Agriculture

In the summer of 1816 there was snow and frost in northern New England and Canada. In both North America and Europe, many crops did not ripen, and in the train of their failure came famine, disease, and social distress. The year 1816 became known as the year without a summer, and climatologists generally attribute the cause to the cataclysmic eruption of Mount Tambora, a volcano in Indonesia, the year before. Tambora spewed out so much ash that, for nearly 400 miles around, the sky was pitch dark for two days. It ejected an estimated 200 million metric tons of fine dust and sulfuric acid, some as high as the stratosphere. The stratospheric veil from this fine debris is probably what robbed the following year of its summer.[3]

The effects of Tambora's eruption are perhaps a mild foretaste of the disruptions to agriculture that might follow a nuclear exchange. Temperature fluctuations can affect crops either by acute, short-term changes, like a sudden frost, or by long-term changes, such as a reduction in average annual temperature. Some crops have a certain resistance to freezing; germinating spring wheat can withstand temperatures down to 9 degrees centigrade below freezing. Others, like rice, die at just below the freezing point. At New Haven, Connecticut, in the year following the Tambora eruption, there were frosts in May, a week of killing frosts in June, and brief nighttime frosts in July and August. Most of the crops that germinated in late May were killed by the June frosts, many crops planted in June died in July, and those that had survived the earlier frosts died in August. Corn production in the region was almost eliminated.

A nuclear war in spring or summer could cause immediate episodes of freezing that might ruin harvests throughout the Northern Hemisphere. A war at any season could wreak havoc with harvests if its dust and smoke veil persisted for many weeks and brought the risk of summer freezes.

Besides promoting freezes, a nuclear smoke shroud would reduce or abolish harvests simply by lowering the annual average temperature. This measure is remarkably constant; the average annual Northern Hemisphere temperature has stayed within plus or minus 0.75 of a degree for the last century. Even a small departure from the average annual temperature can affect a crop's viability. A cooling can squeeze the growing season by inducing freezes later in spring or earlier in fall. This is a particular threat to crops grown at the northern extremities of their natural range. A 1-degree cooling "would nearly eliminate wheat growing in Canada."[4]

Another effect of cooling is to reduce the number of days with temperatures above a certain minimum, thereby decreasing yields. A temperature reduction of 3 degrees centigrade would completely eliminate the growing of wheat in Canada. A 4- to 6-degree reduction in average annual temperature would abolish yields of soybeans in the southern United States.[5]

The effects of a slight cooling are not so straightforward for crops that, unlike Canadian wheat, are grown below the extremities of their range. A cooling of 1 to 2 degrees centigrade would *increase* yields by one to three bushels an acre in the major wheat-producing states of America, according to the National Academy of Sciences, and a warming of 1 to 2 degrees would do the reverse. A 1.5-degree cooling and a 5 percent decrease in precipitation would do wonders for the corn crop in the United States.[6]

But larger drops in temperature would doubtless make it impossible to grow certain crops in their present latitudes. The best available estimates for the kind of temperature drop that might follow a 6,500-megaton war in spring or summer are the following: 15 to 35 degrees below normal for the first few weeks; 5 to 30 degrees for the next one to six months; 0 to 10 degrees for the next few years. These estimates are for the interiors of continents at mid-latitudes in the Northern Hemisphere. At tropical latitudes, the extent of cooling would be 0 to 15 degrees for the first six months, 0 to 5 degrees for the next few years. Temperatures around coastal areas would be very erratic because the warmth from the oceans would vie with cold winds from the interior.

For a war that occurred in winter, the anticipated temperature drops would be lower: in northern mid-latitudes, a drop of between 0 and 20 degrees in the first few weeks, 0 to 15 degrees over the next one to six months, and 0 to 5 degrees for the first few years.[7] What do these coolings mean for agriculture? A group of experts convened by the Scientific Committee on Problems of the Environment concluded that, after acute disturbances in climate from a war in July, "harvest operations in Canada, U.S.S.R., and W. Europe would be severely affected. Cold and darkness would cause maize, soybeans, potatoes, and rice to fail." (In America, India, and China, some winter- and spring-grown cereals would already have been harvested by July.) If major disturbances in climate were to follow a January war, the experts predict, most crops of winter and spring wheat, barley, and corn would fail in North America, the Soviet Union, and China. Rice in Japan and China would fail. Potatoes in the Soviet Union and Europe would produce no yield. Spring-sown soybeans in the southern United States could yield effectively with enough rain.[8]

In short, nuclear winter at any season carries the risk of disrupting and even eliminating many major crops throughout the Northern Hemisphere. With or without nuclear winter, a nuclear war is likely to destroy harvests in the United States and the Soviet Union, affecting all countries that depend on imports of American grain. The effects of nuclear winter are therefore especially relevant to other countries of the Northern Hemisphere, where a nuclear war would not by itself disrupt agricultural production.

Besides the damage from temperature changes, harvests would also be reduced by any failure to supply the fuel, fertilizers, and pesticides on which crops now depend. Modern agriculture requires the support of sophisticated products from the rest of the economy. No one knows what a postwar economy would be like, but should it fail to supply these inputs, the present energy-intensive style of agriculture would lose much of its enormous productivity. Modern crop varieties are bred to respond to heavy doses of fertilizer; without them, yields would drop sharply.

The Threat of Famine

Major reductions in yields would create serious problems for the world's supply of food. The crisis would be worsened by the probable disruption of the normal patterns of distribution and trade. Only a handful of nations have cereals for export—the United States, Canada, countries of the European Common Market, Argentina, and Australia. Climatic effects aside, a nuclear exchange is likely to devastate the economies and agricultural production of all except the two smallest exporters, Argentina and Australia. Countries that depend heavily on imported cereals, like Japan and much of Africa, might quickly run short. Most countries have less than half a year's food supply in storage. The total grain storage in the world is only 40 days' worth of world consumption.

Because of its vast production, the United States has large amounts of food in storage, enough to feed its own population for a year. But even that would be little cause for comfort if the distribution system were to break down for lack of fuel or transport. The northeastern United States, for example, imports 80 percent of its food from other states or abroad. A breakdown of the elaborate systems for processing and storing food would lead to much spoilage and contamination. "Millions would starve to death in the first few years following an all-out nuclear war," according to Alexander Leaf of the Massachusetts General Hospital.[9]

Taking into account climatic disturbances and the disruption of exports, some put the death toll even higher. "It may well be that the greatest effect on humans from a large-scale nuclear war would be famine. Globally, on the order of [a billion] people could die from starvation," writes Mark Harwell of Cornell University.[10]

"Under a scenario containing no climatic alterations, but with loss of imports and high energy subsidies to agriculture, from 60% to 130% of the current population [of 15 sample countries] could be maintained indefinitely," estimates the International Council of Scientific Unions' study of nuclear war.[11] Thus, even without nuclear winter, the disruption of trade and agriculture inputs could cause many to starve throughout the world.

Nuclear Aftereffects and the Environment

A large-scale nuclear exchange would impose many different stresses on the natural environment. Plants and animals far away from the sites of detonation would experience (a) reduced light and temperature from climatic changes, (b) radiation from global fallout, (c) toxins spread by the fires of burning cities, and

(d) increased fluxes of ultraviolet light because of the reduction of the ozone layer.

Predicting how an assemblage of plants and animals would respond to any one of these changes is hard enough; assessing the response to all the changes coming together is even harder. Stresses that might be easily tolerable individually could be overwhelming in concert. Taking the nuclear aftereffects one by one, the following are the major impacts that each might exert on the plants and animals of the natural environment.[12]

Climatic Changes. If the smoke clouds of a nuclear war cause freezing temperatures at the earth's surface, many plants may be killed, particularly if the freeze lasts for more than a few days. Plants at risk include those of temperate latitudes in summertime and of tropical forests. In the forests of the Northern Hemisphere, sudden freezing would make many plants and trees lose all their leaves. Most would survive to the next season unless the freeze were to last for two months or so, in which case most trees would die. Many animals could die from cold and lack of food, and all except migratory birds would perish.

Tropical forests would be devastated by much lesser and briefer temperature drops, since all tropical plants are very sensitive to chilling. A freeze would probably kill parts of the forest above ground. If it lasted for less than a week, some plants could send up new stems or buds. Many tropical animals, being adapted to live in trees, would perish when deprived of the food and cover of the forest.

Mangroves, trees that occupy coastal waters in a wide band to the north and south of the equator, are extremely sensitive to cold. Almost all species would be killed by a sudden freeze. Mangrove swamps are important as breeding grounds for fish and other species and as regulators of the intertidal environment.

Climatic disturbances following a nuclear war could have a

far-reaching effect on marine life. The oceans contain too much heat to be affected even by the chill of a nuclear winter, but the microscopic plants that inhabit the topmost waters would be affected by any prolonged reduction of light. The plants, known as phytoplankton, live at the surface and down to depths where light is attenuated to 1 percent of its surface intensity. The lower-dwelling phytoplankton would find it hard to carry on photosynthesis during a prolonged period of reduced light and would cease to grow. Since the phytoplankton are the basis of many ocean food chains, a widespread loss of photosynthesis could seriously affect the microscopic animals that feed on the phytoplankton, and the fish larvae that feed on these animals, the zooplankton. The plankton would probably recover after light levels returned to normal.

Ultraviolet Light. Light from the ultraviolet region of the spectrum is harmful to living things because it interacts with and damages both the hereditary material, DNA, and the peptide bond, the chemical link that forms the backbone of protein molecules. Were the ultraviolet component of sunlight to reach the earth's surface unimpeded, life might be possible only in the oceans. Ultraviolet light is screened out by the ozone shield high in the stratosphere. Ozone is a gas formed from oxygen by sunlight and destroyed by the ultraviolet light it absorbs. But the ozone shield is also destroyed by other chemicals, including the oxides of nitrogen.

Nuclear weapons, as noted in chapter 7, heat the oxygen and nitrogen of the atmosphere to temperatures at which they react together and form nitrogen oxides. If enough oxides reach high enough, they are likely to speed the destruction of the ozone shield and attenuate it, allowing more ultraviolet light to reach the earth's surface.

Because of the danger of ultraviolet rays, animals and plants have in the course of evolution developed special enzymes that repair the breakages in chains of DNA caused by ultraviolet light. The thickness of the ozone shield waxes and wanes for natural reasons, and the extra ultraviolet light let through during these fluctuations is generally not harmful. Sunburn and certain skin cancers caused by overexposure to sunlight are an exception. Nuclear war might allow larger than usual fluxes of ultraviolet light to penetrate the ozone shield. In the aftermath of a nuclear exchange, the dust and smoke would act as a substitute shield, but these would vanish in months and it might take years for the ozone shield to re-form.

Enhanced ultraviolet light reduces photosynthesis in plants and so might limit crop yields. Heavy exposure can damage the eyes of animals that do not take steps to protect themselves. Humans could always wear sunglasses, if available, but animals that are unable to convert to nocturnal habits could suffer retinal damage and, in time, blindness.

An increase in ultraviolet light would raise the incidence of skin cancer. Another effect in humans, possibly of considerable importance in the aftermath of nuclear war, is the depression of the immune system.

The extent of all these effects is difficult to predict. High-yield warheads, which loft large amounts of nitrogen oxides to the level of the stratosphere, could reduce the ozone shield substantially. Both superpowers, the United States in particular, are shifting toward warheads of smaller yield as their missiles become more accurate. The danger of ozone depletion diminishes as this trend progresses, but the soot of nuclear winter might increase the risk.

Tropospheric Ozone. While the ozone shield in the stratosphere would be depleted by nuclear war, small amounts of ozone might be created in the lower atmosphere. Ozone is a potent poison for plants, and the minute quantities present in the normal atmosphere cause considerable damage to crops and forests. Rising ozone levels produced by industrial and auto pollution may be contributing to the death of forests in Europe and to extensive crop losses in the eastern United States. The copious nitrogen oxides created in a nuclear exchange could continue to catalyze the formation of extra ozone for months afterward, with corresponding effects on vegetation.

Pyrotoxins. The cities set ablaze in a nuclear exchange would produce not only smoke and soot but also a range of noxious chemicals, some of which might have long-term effects on the environment. Combustion of the certain common city materials is likely to produce the highly toxic chemicals known as dioxins and furans. The destruction of buildings would liberate copious amounts of asbestos, which can cause lung cancer, and of PCBs, the toxic chemical used as an insulator in electrical equipment.

If spread evenly over large areas, all of these potent poisons would be so diluted as to present no major threat to human health. The chances are, however, that they will not be evenly dispersed. Rainfall washing them down could create local hot spots with higher concentrations. All these substances are slow-acting poisons, so their effect might not be recognized until too late. They are also very slow to degrade in the environment.

Radiation. Radioactive fallout, as noted in chapter 4, is usually considered in two categories—local and global. Local fallout is that deposited downwind during the first one or two days after a detonation. Fallout trails can extend for several hundred miles from ground zero; in a major exchange, a significant part of the land surface of the United States could be covered with local fallout. In the highest concentrations of a fallout zone, radiation reaches levels lethal to humans, who are among the most sensitive of animals, and to certain plants, like conifers.

Global fallout is a much less serious threat. Carried on fine particles that remain suspended for weeks or months, the radioactivity is dispersed around the globe before settling, and also has longer to decay before reaching the ground. The highest dose of global fallout from a major exchange is likely to be less than 40 rads in the Northern Hemisphere. The LD-50 for humans (the dose that will kill half of a population exposed to it) is generally assumed to be 450 rads, and a 40-rad dose is of little immediate concern.

On the other hand, the global fallout may become concentrated—for example, in localities with heavy rainfall—building up to harmful levels. It may also become concentrated in the food chain. From nuclear tests conducted in the atmosphere, it is known that lichens absorb radioactive particles from the air, accumulating considerably higher doses than do the plants around them. Reindeer and caribou that graze on the lichens absorb the radioactivity in their bodies. Radioactivity has been detected in the Lapps who fed on the reindeer and in the Eskimos who ate the caribou.

The immediate threat of radioactivity is from external doses to the body. But people who lived in a radioactively contaminated environment, eating contaminated food and water, would soon begin to accumulate radioactivity in their bodies. They would then receive an internal dose that can be much more harmful. Certain kinds of radiation, known as alpha and beta radiation, are stopped by clothes or at the skin surface, and pose little threat as external doses. But once the emitting atoms become lodged in the body's organs, the alpha and beta radiation is absorbed internally and may cause serious damage. Plutonium, for example, is a strong and long-lived emitter of alpha radiation. If plutonium dust is breathed in, a particle may lodge in the lung or enter the bloodstream and be deposited in the liver or bone. Continuous exposure of these organs to the short-range but energetic alpha particles may cause cancer.

From low external doses of global fallout, plants and animals may concentrate radioactivity in food chains and accumulate significant internal doses.

Within the areas of local fallout, the high radiation levels will damage plants and animals according to each species' susceptibility to radiation. Mammals and birds are the most sensitive to radiation; insects are comparatively resistant. Plants also vary widely in sensitivity, the difference being connected with the size of their chromosomes at a certain stage of cell division. Pines and other conifers can be damaged or killed at much the same levels that kill humans; most other plants are more resistant. Viruses and bacteria have the most resistance of all.

Within a local fallout zone, insects and bacteria are likely to be far less affected than pinewoods and humans. They will start with a competitive advantage in the process of recovery.

Concurrent Stresses. Unless climatic changes are severe, causing freezes that kill plants throughout the Northern Hemisphere, few of the effects described above are likely to be of immediate danger to plants or animals. But each is a stress to living things, and the cumulative burden could be more serious than expected. Plants could well survive the stresses of reduced sunlight, increased ultraviolet light, a few rads of radiation, and noxious gases when exposed to each separately, but they might be less adaptable in dealing with several simultaneously. The human immune system is depressed by radiation, by ultraviolet light, and by malnutrition. The three stresses acting in concert might seriously sap the survivors' resistance to disease although this is a matter of conjecture.

9

Casualties and Survivors

Even a small nuclear attack, limited to a handful of weapons, would be an unparalleled disaster for the United States or the Soviet Union. Yet there is considerable reason to estimate the results of different kinds of nuclear war because of the very different outcome for the survivors. Barring ecological catastrophe, the United States and the Soviet Union are likely to make an economic recovery from attacks confined to military targets. But after a nuclear war involving cities and industrial centers, the possibility of recovery would hang in the balance.

No one knows what targets in the other's territory each superpower would select for nuclear attack. Nuclear strategists sometimes assume that a nuclear war would occur in stages, starting with a "counterforce" duel in which each side tried first to take out the other's strategic nuclear weapons. Or an attacker might include industrial as well as strategic targets so as to impede postwar economic recovery. This is termed a countervalue attack. There is military logic in threatening cities, but none in hitting them, unless they contain strategic or industrial targets. Nevertheless, many cities do include or lie near such targets.

Official American doctrine holds that a nuclear attack on the

United States will be met with "flexible response." This means that a nuclear attack with a few weapons will be answered not with massive retaliation but with enough weapons to deter the aggressor from further escalation. The objective is to halt a nuclear war at the lowest possible level of destruction. By refraining from destroying the opponent's cities, the doctrine teaches, each side will hope to earn the reciprocal restraint that will protect its own. Many analysts doubt, however, that a nuclear war, once started, could be contained at any level below an all-out exchange.

The question of casualties in a nuclear war has recently been reviewed by the Office of Technology Assessment (OTA), a research arm of Congress. One case considered by the OTA is that of counterforce attacks by the United States and the Soviet Union against one another. Such attacks are confined to strategic nuclear forces, including missiles, bombers, submarines, and the nuclear command structures that control them. Another is that of an all-out attack on military and industrial targets.[1]

Consequences of a Counterforce Attack

A counterforce attack by the Soviet Union would presumably target American missile silos and their control centers, bomber bases and missile submarine support bases. The salvo of warheads blitzing the main missile silos sites in the Great Plains would kill relatively few people directly but would create massive amounts of radioactive fallout. Depending on the prevailing winds, the fallout would be carried for hundreds of miles, probably in an easterly direction, and would blanket thousands of square miles in the Great Lakes region and the Northeast with lethal amounts of radioactivity. Most submarine ports and bomber bases are near large cities, and at each target hundreds of thousands of people might be killed instantly.

The number of casualties from such an attack could vary widely. Warheads exploded at or near the earth's surface create considerable fallout; airbursts produce little or none. The distribution of fallout depends critically on wind, which disperses it, and on rain, which washes out the radioactive particles and produces concentrated zones of high radiation. Existing fallout shelters, if used, would provide effective protection for many citizens.

Depending on the assumptions made about these various factors, casualty estimates differ widely. From a review of several government studies of nuclear counterforce attacks, the OTA concludes that the likely number of deaths could range from 1 to 20 million people. The low estimate assumes no surface bursts, good protection from fallout, and abnormally light winds, so that most radioactivity falls back at the site of the detonation. The high estimate assumes that there is no crisis period preceding the attack and no opportunity to advise citizens on how to protect against fallout.

Most of the government studies estimate that the number of injured would be about the same as the number of deaths. All include both immediate deaths and those occurring up to 30 days after an attack. One estimate of Soviet casualties from an American counterforce attack is that 4 to 14 million would die.

These government figures are based on extrapolations from the numbers killed by blast at Hiroshima and may underestimate the number of people who would die in the fires created by larger weapons. At Hiroshima the weapon's yield was so small—a mere 12.5 kilotons—that the blast wave killed people throughout a larger area than did the fires set by the thermal pulse. With the one-megaton (1,000 kiloton) weapons that are now common in both sides' strategic arsenals, the superfires (discussed in chapter 3) would cover a larger area than the lethal blast wave. The fires might reach out from 5 to 9.3 miles (8 to 15 kilometers) from ground zero, depending on visibility and other factors. The afterwinds following a one-megaton explosion would last much longer and therefore do more damage than those of the Hiroshima bomb. Except from the outer ring of the fire zone, few people would be able to escape through streets blocked with fire debris and reamed with hurricane force winds.

The effect of superfires has been noted in a new casualty estimate by William Daugherty, Barbara Levi, and Frank von Hippel of Princeton University.[2] Because the fires would kill many of those assumed in the government studies to be merely injured, the Princeton group finds that rather more people would be killed outright and fewer would be left injured. They estimate that a counterforce attack on the United States would cause 20 million immediate deaths and 26 million injured.

All government estimates and the Princeton figures quoted above are based on the assumption that deaths from radiation occur at the lethal dose, or LD-50/60, of 450 rads. (The LD-50/60 is the dose that will kill half of the people exposed to it within 60 days; a rad is a standard unit of radiation.) This value for the LD-50/60 may overestimate the hardiness of humans to radiation. In a study conducted in 1960 it was argued that among a population denied antibiotics and blood transfusions, the standard treatment for radiation sickness, the LD-50 would be as low 350 rads. As discussed in chapter 5, the LD-50 for the inhabitants of Hiroshima may have been as little as 220 rads. But as the author of this study points out, this value for the LD-50 relates to wartime conditions. American and Soviet populations are far healthier, and would be expected to have greater initial resistance to radiation, than Japanese debilitated by years of war. Nonetheless, the LD-50 might well prove to be lower than the current estimate of 450 rads. If it were as low as 350 rads, the Princeton group estimates, there would be an extra 2 to 3 million deaths and 3 to 6 million injured in a counterforce attack on the United States.

Casualties from a Nuclear Countervalue Attack

Nuclear war might begin as an outright attack against military and industrial targets. Or a war that began just as a counterforce attack might escalate to a countervalue attack. The casualties in a countervalue attack would be considerably greater. According to government studies surveyed by the OTA, estimates of American fatalities from a Soviet countervalue attack range from a maximum of between 155 million and 165 million deaths to a minimum of between 20 million and 55 million. These fatalities are for the first 30 days following the attack and do not include later deaths among the injured or from economic disruption and deprivation.

For Soviet deaths from an American countervalue attack, estimates range from a maximum of 64 to 100 million, to a minimum of between 50 and 80 million. In both the American and Soviet cases, the difference between the high and low estimates depends on such factors as whether the population has time to evacuate target areas and what types and yields of weapon are used in the attack.

Recovery after Nuclear War

The extent of recovery after a nuclear exchange depends considerably on the nature of an attack. A counterforce attack, by definition, is not aimed at crippling the economic production of a country. Although enormous collateral damage would be sustained, the economic basis for reconstruction would still exist. But recovery would hang in the balance after a countervalue attack, the purpose of which is to destroy economic targets.

After a counterforce attack people living in zones contaminated with radioactivity would have to stay in shelters. Others also would probably stay in shelters or evacuated areas until reassured that no further attacks were likely. During this period, which would last at least a month from the initial attack, most economic activity would cease.

In the view of the OTA, there is little doubt that an economic recovery would successfully be made after a counterforce nuclear attack. "Economic viability would not be at issue following a counterforce attack. Because the attack seeks no economic damage, it would be far less likely than a deliberate strike on economic targets to create any bottlenecks that would greatly hinder recovery. The Nation would be able to restore production and maintain self-sufficiency. The attack would cause enormous economic loss, but the Nation's capacity for growth would be at worst only slightly impaired."

A principal problem in the recovery would be agriculture, since millions of acres in the Great Plains would be contaminated with fallout, preventing farmers from working the fields. Another problem would be the decontaminating of cities, farms, and factories of radioactivity. The bulldozer and firehose crews that moved the fallout would doubtless have to expose themselves to considerable amounts of radiation. Public health standards would have to be relaxed as the assumption of such risks became necessary.

The degree of economic disorganization might be severe. "Once people were confident that the war had ended," the OTA report notes, "money would retain its value, and so would property in uncontaminated areas. But the marketplace that organizes the American economy would be severely disrupted by abrupt shifts in demand, abrupt changes in supply, questions about the validity of contracts involving people or things in contaminated areas. . . ."

The Soviet Union, too, would certainly recover from a counterforce attack, in the OTA's view. Its system of central planning might in some respects be better adapted to the exigencies of recovery, since it would be less affected by the disruption of money, credit, and contracts that might paralyze a market economy.

A countervalue attack on the United States would cause a different magnitude of disorder. The far greater destruction of people and physical resources would deeply erode the basis of economic recovery. Nonetheless, though physical assets would be severely reduced, there would be fewer people in need of them. The survivors might at first be able to live off the remaining stocks of goods without meeting any particular shortages, with the probable exception of medicines.

But once the interim stockpiles were exhausted, the OTA report argues, new production might have considerable difficulty in filling requirements. Production in the United States is a complex process of many stages and different levels of organization. These require an organized work force and elaborate systems of transport and communications. Unless law and order remain intact, people will be unwilling to leave the security of their homes. If surviving assets were not evenly distributed, regional disparities might emerge, followed by regional conflicts. If money were replaced with barter, a highly inefficient means of exchange, the surviving resources would not be used to best advantage.

A critical point would soon be reached at which the prewar inventories of goods started to give out. If by that stage new means of production were not on hand to replace them, the economy would be headed inexorably toward regression and collapse. In effect, notes the OTA, "The country would enter a race with economic viability as the prize. The country would try to restore production to the point where consumption of stocks and the wearing out of surviving goods and tools was matched by new production. If this was achieved before stocks ran out, then viability would be attained. Otherwise, consumption would necessarily sink to the level of new production and in so doing would probably depress production further, creating a downward spiral. At some point this spiral would stop, but by the time it did so the United States might have returned to the economic equivalent of the Middle Ages."

Recovery in the Soviet Union would also hang in the balance after a countervalue nuclear attack. The destruction of cities, where most Russians live, might tip the balance of power toward other nationalities. But enough party members would survive that the government would probably be able to maintain control. Because of the inefficiencies of central planning, however, surviving resources would not be well used, and production would go down before it went up. If things went well, government organization and brute force methods could overcome production bottlenecks, providing enough production to sustain survivors in food, housing, and medical care. If things went badly, harvests would be lost, transportation would collapse, Eastern Europe would revolt, and neighbors like China might threaten invasion causing resources to be diverted to war. Should economic production collapse for such reasons, fewer people could be supported. The Soviet Union's failure to achieve economic viability could cause as many deaths as the nuclear attack.

Falling Back on the Environment

The prospects for economic recovery discussed by the OTA report of 1979 do not take account of nuclear winter, an effect discovered later. The likely extent of a nuclear winter is still a matter of keen debate. What if it were fully as bad as feared?

According to some biologists, nuclear winter would be so harsh as to disrupt agriculture altogether. Surviving groups of humans would be obliged to live in the wild, hunting and gathering berries as humankind did in Paleolithic times. Natural ecosystems could probably provide subsistence for only 1 percent of the world's five billion people, and for even less of percentage if the natural environment were severely degraded by the aftereffects of nuclear war.

Even if the natural environment recovers from a nuclear exchange, some foresee a future for human societies that is even bleaker than that predicted by the OTA. According to Alexander Leaf, "So much of the social and economic structure of society as we know it would be destroyed that relationships which we take for granted would disappear. Money would have little or no value. Food and other necessities would be obtained, when available, by barter. More likely, as people became desperate with hunger, survival instincts would take over and armed individuals or marauding bands would raid and pilfer what supplies and stores existed. Those fortunates who had stores would hoard their resources and soon become the victims of the crazed behavior of starving and desperate survivors who would ransack warehouses and attack individual homes. Law enforcement would not exist and many would be killed in the fighting between those trying forcefully to obtain possession of food stores and those trying to protect their own homes, families, and food supplies."[3]

Given the probability that the telephone grid will have been disrupted by nuclear electromagnetic pulses and communications been destroyed, many regions could be isolated. Authority might break down and severe disorder appear in the immediate aftermath of a nuclear exchange.

"If 50 percent or more of the populations of the belligerent countries are destroyed, the result could be the end of these particular societies or civilizations as we know them," writes the economist Yves Laulan. He believes that money would be replaced by barter, that investment would disappear because all remaining production would be devoted to procuring basic needs, and that trade would cease. The result would be "the total disappearance of organized large and medium scale economic activity at both the national and international levels. . . . Many activities we now take for granted would simply disappear. There would be an extraordinary drop in the resources available for consumption, which would precipitate an instantaneous drop in the standard of living. It might be like going from the 20th

Century back to the dark ages at the snap of a finger. We would be reduced to bare subsistence, and it is clear that this situation would continue for a long time." As for political structure, Laulan thinks that the struggle for survival would dictate the emergence of authoritarian societies, based on agriculture and independent of one another.[4]

However devastating a nuclear exchange, Laulan's predictions are open to question. The so-called Dark Ages were allegedly characterized by a lack of enlightenment, and knowledge is not destroyed by nuclear weapons. Germany and Japan after World War II endured the devastation of most of their major cities, with massive civilian and military casualties. The survivors, despite the demoralization of defeat, retained their skills and memory of what their societies had been; their urge was to rebuild, and the economic success of postwar Germany and Japan is well known.

But prospects for a postnuclear United States and Soviet Union would be far less favorable. Allied bombing of Germany destroyed residential areas in city centers but left the factories in the suburbs largely unscathed. Japan's wrecked economy benefited from American aid and the Korean War's stimulus to demand. Both Germany and Japan, note Hal Cochrane and Dennis Mileti, were favored by special factors: "No nation would have the resources or possibly the will to come to the aid of a United States devastated by a nuclear exchange. Food stuffs would be hoarded rather than shared. No world wide economic boom would ensue. Without an external source of demand for its products, the U.S. economy would languish."[5]

A large-scale nuclear exchange would be more destructive than even World War II, and its social and economic impact would be the more devastating for being applied in perhaps a single day rather than over five or more years. Postwar Europe arose from exhaustion because of American economic aid delivered through the Marshall Plan. In a postnuclear world, there might be no benefactors with resources to spare, and no Marshall Plan to assist the devastated nuclear powers.

Even if the natural environment were seriously deranged or degraded, as it might well be, steps cannot be retraced in history; there is no question of turning the clock back or returning to a more primitive epoch of civilization. But the complexity of contemporary economies and the highly educated populations that run them make for intricate organizations that are easily shattered and hard to put back together. To repair the havoc of a nuclear exchange lasting an afternoon might take the work of generations. Building a new, postnuclear world would not necessarily be impossible. But the old world would be beyond healing.

10

Rethinking
Nuclear War

In the last ten years a series of discoveries have been made about the consequences of nuclear weapons, culminating in that of the nuclear winter effect. As the details have been filled in, the portrait of nuclear war has grown even more repugnant and unacceptable. There is now an evident possibility that an extensive nuclear war would devastate the natural environment far more severely than ever supposed. This new understanding prompts a reexamination of the policy of nuclear deterrence. Yet many nuclear strategists who have discussed nuclear winter conclude that it only confirms the desirability of present policies. How can that be? And if it be, is there not some flaw in their basic assumptions?

Nuclear strategy, perhaps surprisingly, is an esoteric subject. It is dominated by a tiny coterie of specialists who have debated the subject so finely as to turn it into an abstruse doctrine, bristling with paradox and tests of faith. Yet this doctrine has become the declared policy of the United States. In its terms, high officials seek to explain to the public why the government must possess and keep on building a panoply of weapons so terrible they can never be used.

For nuclear strategists, nuclear winter is the incarnation of an idea they debated thirty years ago—the doomsday machine of Herman Kahn. The machine was to consist of a computer connected to an arsenal of nuclear weapons, enough to blanket the world in lethal fallout. The computer would fire the weapons as soon as it sensed the Soviet Union had committed some act defined as intolerable. Kahn invented the doomsday concept to satirize the nuclear policy of massive destruction that then prevailed. The strategists' ideas on how to avoid triggering the doomsday machine have become official policy, espoused in one form or another by Administrations of the last 20 years.

Nuclear winter suggests some possibly desirable modifications to present policy, notably in the design and fusing of warheads, target selection, ballistic missile defense, and approaches to arms control. But far from overturning present policy, nuclear winter—in the strategists' view—reaffirms its central dogma: that in case deterrence fails, it is preferable to have options that allow for war to be terminated short of total destruction.

The Structure of Nuclear Deterrence

Anyone who looks for the first time at the nuclear forces maintained by the superpowers is likely to be appalled at their apparent excess. A single nuclear weapon detonated over a capital city might be thought enough to deter any rational leaders from aggression. Yet the United States and the Soviet Union each possess about 10,000 strategic nuclear weapons, deliverable from land, sea, and air, and a total of about 50,000 devices if "tactical" nuclear weapons are also included. The firing of even a few weapons risks triggering the complete launching of both arsenals. How did the stockpiles of nuclear weapons grow so large? What assumptions justify their deployment?

Nuclear arsenals are sometimes criticized, among other things, for their expense. The reality is the opposite. Nuclear weapons, however expensive in absolute terms, have always been cheap in comparison with the perceived alternative—vast standing armies. The United States and its European allies do not lack the manpower or resources to raise conventional armies of the same size as the Soviet Union's. Rather than put their economies on a wartime footing, they have consistently chosen to maintain smaller armies supplemented by nuclear weapons.

This policy began almost immediately after the Second World War, when American armies were demobilized and sent home from Europe but the Red Army remained in possession of Eastern Europe. In the Cold War that soon ensued, both superpowers continued to develop nuclear weapons and their means of delivery. By 1949 the United States possessed almost 300 nuclear bombs.

Two international events, in particular, stimulated major expansions of each side's nuclear forces. The experience of the Korean War persuaded American policymakers that the United States could not easily afford its gross disadvantage in manpower compared with that of the Soviet Union and the People's Republic of China. President Eisenhower, declining to raise taxes or run large deficits, saw increased nuclear forces as an affordable means of bolstering national defense and maintaining American strategic superiority.

President Kennedy reaped the success of this policy in the Cuban missile crisis of October 1962. A local advantage in conventional forces and a global superiority in strategic weapons enabled him to secure the withdrawal of Soviet missiles from Cuba. But the Soviet Union drew the lesson that it must obtain strategic parity or better in order to avoid similar reverses in future. It began a major expansion of its strategic forces, building large numbers of land-based missiles and, following the United States, a force of missile-carrying submarines.

For independent reasons in its historical experience, each side thus has motives for maintaining large strategic forces. There are also interdependent reasons. Each superpower was the victim of an attack it did not expect in the Second World War, and each strives continually to protect against a surprise nuclear attack from the other. The smaller the number of missiles and warheads, the greater the risk that an adversary might be able to destroy all of them.

The danger is even more acute. A nation need not disable all its opponent's nuclear forces in order to deliver a disarming blow; it only has to destroy enough of them to discourage the opponent from retaliating. Therefore each side strives to maintain such a superabundance of nuclear forces that it could ride out a first strike and still possess enough weapons to devastate the aggressor.

Assured Destruction and Flexible Response

Another pressure toward the formation of large arsenals of nuclear weapons comes from the doctrine that governs how they are to be used. Since the Second World War, strategic thinking has veered between the two objectives sometimes known as assured destruction and flexible response. Assured destruction, the devastation of an opponent's society, can be accomplished with relatively few weapons. Flexible response requires the weapons to provide a whole series of nuclear options, from which the President may select a response appropriate to the initial aggression. The doctrine envisages the possibility of a series of steps in nuclear war, at each of which attempts might be made to negotiate and conclude the war. The theory is to deter an opponent at some level of nuclear violence short of massive destruction of each other's cities.[1]

From the generally unsuccessful record of precision strategic bombing in the Second World War, many Air Force commanders drew the lesson that destruction of large, easily hit targets like cities was the only kind of bombing campaign likely to be effective. American targeting policy was initially based on the concept of massive destruction and the thesis that a nuclear war could be fought and won like other wars. In a speech of January 1954, Secretary of State John Foster Dulles declared that American policy would be to respond to local aggression with "the further deterrent of massive retaliatory power." The doctrine of Dulles's "massive retaliation" speech grew from a situation in which the United States possessed strategic nuclear superiority yet lacked the conventional forces to fight in Korea and to counter a feared Soviet thrust in Europe. The first Single Integrated Operational Plan, approved in 1960, called for an all-out attack on the Soviet Union in which 4,000 weapons were to be fired in a single spasm.

The Strategic Air Command's policy of massive destruction was opposed from the start by civilian analysts employed at RAND, the Air Force's think tank. Humanitarian objections aside, the RAND analysts argued it was preferable to hold cities hostage than to destroy them, especially since destruction of an opponent's cities would invite retaliation against one's own. In a circumstance where nuclear weapons had to be used, a measured response against military targets, with worse held in reserve, might persuade the Soviets to desist and negotiate without escalating the level of violence.

This doctrine, which came to be known as Flexible Response, embraces the idea that attacks on an opponent's nuclear weapons (counterforce) and military-industrial capacity (countervalue) are preferable to attacks on cities, which should be held as targets of last resort. Concepts of counterforce won a sympathetic hearing from Secretary of Defense Robert McNamara. Nonetheless McNamara, largely to fix an upper limit to American strategic nuclear forces for domestic political and budgetary reasons, enunciated the doctrine of Assured Destruction, "the capability to destroy the aggressor as a viable society, even after a well-planned and executed surprise attack on our forces."

President Nixon reemphasized flexibility. He said in 1971, "I must not be—and my successors must not be—limited to the indiscriminate mass destruction of enemy civilians as the sole possible response to challenges. We must ensure that we have the forces and procedures that provide us with alternatives appropriate to the nature and the level of the provocation."

The weakness of the doctrine of nuclear deterrence has always been what to do if deterrence should fail. The strategists' answer is: first, strengthen deterrence yet further and second, prepare to fight a nuclear war at all levels up to massive destruction in the hope that war can be contained at the lowest. The logic of the argument dictates building nuclear weapons capable of destroying military targets, like missiles in hardened silos, as well as the command and control apparatus the enemy needs to assess damage and move to the next level of nuclear violence— in other words, the ability to fight a nuclear war.

Nuclear war fighting, in the strategists' view, is critical to deterrence. Suppose a Soviet attack is concentrated on American nuclear forces, leaving cities unharmed. If the President's only option is to destroy Soviet society with his remaining forces, the Soviets will retaliate against American cities. The United States would do better to surrender. But that situation would only encourage a Soviet attack in the first place. If assured destruction is the President's only option, the credibility of deterrence is eroded. *Si vis pacem, para bellum;* to deter a nuclear war, prepare to fight one.

At the time of President Nixon's statement, the American strategic plan contained only a few attack options, each requiring many hundreds of nuclear weapons. A major review of targeting policy began, culminating in a strategy set forth by Secretary of Defense James Schlesinger, a RAND alumnus. The Schlesinger doctrine, promulgated in a document known as NSDM-242, included limited nuclear options employing just a handful of weapons, a secure reserve force, and a postwar objective of impeding Soviet recovery. The goal was to enable the United States, even after a large nuclear war, to reconstitute itself more rapidly than the Soviet Union.

American forces were at the time incapable of executing the

Schlesinger doctrine. The command and control system was so vulnerable that the President would not have had assured control over the reserve force that survived an initial attack. President Carter came into office talking about reducing the number of nuclear weapons to zero. His secretary of defense, Harold Brown, was skeptical of strategies for winning a nuclear war, considering them impractical: "I remain highly skeptical that escalation of a limited nuclear exchange can be controlled, or that it can be stopped short of an all-out massive exchange." Yet Brown came to realize, as had McNamara before him, that having options is better than having no options. President Carter issued two nuclear strategy documents, PD-18 and PD-59, which endorsed the Schlesinger doctrine and called for procurement of the hardware to implement it. This included, in particular, the MX missile, a weapon that carries ten accurate warheads capable of destroying war-fighting targets, such as Soviet land-based missiles. In PD-59, the ideas developed by the RAND analysts over the preceding 30 years finally came to fruition.

President Reagan has continued the Carter strategy, together with the counterforce weapons it requires, and a more capable command and control system for fighting a nuclear war should deterrence fail. Present American nuclear policy has been summarized by Secretary of Defense Caspar Weinberger: "If deterrence should fail, we cannot predict the nature of a Soviet nuclear strike nor ensure with any certainty that what might begin as a limited Soviet attack would remain confined to that level. We must plan for flexibility in our forces and in our options for response, so that we might terminate the conflict on terms favorable to the forces of freedom, and reestablish deterrence at the lowest possible level of violence, thus avoiding further destruction. . . .

"Maintaining a stable strategic deterrent requires a multiplicity of retaliatory strategic forces—a triad of land-based missiles, manned bombers, and submarine-launched ballistic missiles. The unique characteristics of the independent and separate components that make up the triad bolster deterrence by acting in concert to complicate Soviet attack planning, making it more difficult for the Soviet Union to plan and execute a successful attack on all these components. . . . In addition to a strong triad, stability of deterrence in a crisis and the effective and responsible use of our nuclear forces depend on a response and survivable command, control and communications system."[2]

By their glib pronouncements about nuclear war, some senior officials have given the impression that the Reagan Administration has embarked on a new and more bellicose nuclear strategy. In the event of a nuclear attack, according to Deputy Under Secretary of Defense T. K. Jones, Americans should "dig a hole, cover it with a couple of doors and then throw three feet of dirt on top. . . . If there are enough shovels to go around, everybody's going to make it."[3] In fact, the Reagan Administration added little new to nuclear doctrine except to continue procurement of the hardware needed to implement the Carter strategy. It has made a major change in research, however, by resurrecting the concept of ballistic missile defense. The Strategic Defense Initiative propounded by President Reagan in 1983 is at present only a research and demonstration program but will constitute a major departure in strategic structure if the decision is ever taken to deploy a nationwide missile defense.

Nuclear War Fighting and First Strike Weapons

In the name of being able to fight a nuclear war should deterrence fail, the United States is developing a new generation of weapons capable of destroying Soviet strategic nuclear missiles and command posts. These include the land-based MX and Midgetman missiles, the D5 missile to be carried aboard Trident submarines, the B1-B and Stealth bombers, and air-breathing, cruise missiles launchable from submarines and bombers. These weapons are in part a response to the large Soviet land-based missiles, the SS-18 and SS-19, which during the 1970s gained for the first time a combination of yield and accuracy sufficient to threaten all American land-based missiles.

When the strategic land-based missile forces were invulnerable, the incentive for either side to launch a nuclear attack was greatly reduced. (Submarine-based missiles are still invulnerable, but they have the accuracy only to hit cities, which would provoke retaliation in kind.) The Soviet Union was the first nation to acquire the capacity to destroy the opponent's force of land-based missiles, upsetting the balance. The advance of technology probably made such a development inevitable unless restrained by arms control agreements. That opportunity was missed, and both sides are now rapidly refining their capacity to threaten each other's strategic forces. This destabilizes the strategic balance by encouraging each side, in crisis, to use its forces or lose them.

Land-based ballistic missiles like the MX can quickly knock out the opponent's missiles, a property known as prompt, hard-target kill capability. Bombers and cruise missiles can also destroy missile silos, but not so promptly. The ability to destroy missiles quickly is justified by the Administration as essential to its nuclear war-fighting capability, should deterrence fail.

Strategic Parity, Strategic Superiority, and Arms Control

The United States and the Soviet Union have signed three major agreements setting restraints on strategic nuclear arms. These are the SALT I and Anti-Ballistic Missile treaties of 1972 and the SALT II treaty of 1979. Under the ABM treaty each side agreed not to build defenses against ballistic missiles, except for a single site defense in each country. The SALT II treaty, which supersedes SALT I, sets limits on the numbers of strategic missiles in various categories that each side may deploy.

The basis of the treaty regime was strategic parity, since each side agreed to the same numerical limits. Proponents of the treaties regard them as the foundation for restraining, and ultimately reversing, the race in strategic arms. The only way the Soviet Union could have been induced to accept such restraints, proponents assert, was on the basis of equality in nuclear arms. But critics opposed, among other things, the underlying concept of yielding parity in nuclear arms to the Soviet Union when the United States, in their view, was the inferior in conventional arms. Because of such objections, and the Soviet invasion of Afghanistan, the SALT II treaty has not been ratified by the U.S. Senate. President Reagan observed the treaty during his first five years in office, until Thanksgiving Day 1986, then permitted the treaty's limits to be overstepped.

The SALT treaties, commitments of foreign policy, failed to resolve the domestic debate between those who believe America must retain or regain the nuclear superiority it enjoyed throughout the 1950s and those who believe superiority is a dangerous and unobtainable objective, pursuit of which will only prolong the superpowers' competition in nuclear armaments. The latter tend to see the new generation of prompt, hard-target weapons as potential implements of a first strike, designed to regain nuclear superiority. Those who favor a strong deterrent argue that the more forcefully the Soviet Union is deterred from resorting to nuclear weapons, the less likely is the outbreak of nuclear war.

Nuclear Winter, Nuclear Strategy

American nuclear strategy has evolved over some 40 years of intellectual analysis and political debate. How does the concept of nuclear winter affect this edifice? According to Michael May, a former director of the Lawrence Livermore National Laboratory, "The necessity of avoiding nuclear war already dominates

U.S. and Soviet interactions. The presence or absence of global climatic effects is not likely to change the current balance of judgments, politics and bureaucratic constraints that result in the two sides' pattern of actions."[4] "We are already well persuaded that nuclear war should be deterred. When you ask what the policy implications are, the question is: Are we going to alter our policies, our policies of deterrence? . . . I think the answer to that is no." So Richard Perle, assistant secretary of defense for international security policy, told the Senate Armed Services Committee in an October 1985 hearing devoted to the consequences of nuclear winter.

Perle in essence argued that, albeit for other reasons, the Administration was already doing everything feasible to reduce the likelihood of nuclear winter. It was strengthening deterrence. It was reducing the yield of nuclear warheads. It was committed to a doctrine of not targeting cities. In arms talks with the Soviet Union, it had proposed a major reduction in nuclear warheads. It was pursuing research on methods to destroy Soviet missiles and warheads before detonation.

The one thing the Administration did not propose to do, Perle said, was to shrink arsenals to a size at which the President's only option after a Soviet strike would be to retaliate against cities. He told Senator Sam Nunn of Georgia, "The way to prevent nuclear winter is to prevent nuclear war. The way, in my judgment, to prevent nuclear war is to have an adequate deterrence. That is where I part company with most of the community that has become concerned about nuclear winter because they are, as far as I can tell, deeply committed to mutual assured destruction. . . . That is, reduce the arsenals very substantially and still have enough to destroy the other side. That, Senator, is my understanding of what we are trying to get away from."[5]

Winterizing Nuclear Forces

Though the strategists see no reason to change present doctrine because of nuclear winter, they have several ideas for avoiding the consequences of nuclear winter, should the possibility of the effect be verified. One is to ignore military targets that are located in cities unless they are of extreme importance. Another is to accelerate the trend toward warheads of lower yield and higher accuracy. Ballistic missile warheads cannot change or correct course after being released from their "bus," thousands of miles away from their targets. A new kind of weapon has been developed that can scan the ground for its target as it reenters the atmosphere and maneuver toward it. Such devices, known as maneuvering reentry vehicles, are capable of very high accuracy and so need a considerably smaller explosive yield to destroy their target.

Maneuvering reentry vehicles are already incorporated in the new tactical Pershing-2 missile and are claimed to have an accuracy of 40 meters. Equipped with such warheads, the next generation of strategic missiles could also have significantly smaller yields or perhaps even carry nonnuclear explosives. This would reduce the amount of smoke created and the initial height to which the fireball would carry it.

Another approach is to develop warheads capable of penetrating the ground before detonation. The heat and blast from an earth-penetrating, one-kiloton warhead would ignite fires over an area of less than a hundredth of a square mile.[6] The smoke would be lofted less high, increasing the chance of its being rained out before the sun's heat made it rise to the stratosphere. By contrast, a one-megaton warhead burst above a city might burn out an area of about 175 square miles.

With target changes and the redesign of nuclear warheads, it may well be technically possible to avoid the danger of triggering nuclear winter effects. "Both short and long term effects of such weapons would be dramatically curtailed, and the danger of the ignition of fires virtually eliminated, by a combination of weapons selection and careful targeting," is one forecast.[7] On the other hand, the ground-penetrating warheads would create copious local fallout, since the radioactivity of the nuclear materials and bomb casing would mingle with the earth's debris. Much of the radiating debris would be in the form of heavy particles that would fall out close to the blast area, emitting radiation doses as high as 10,000 rads, or enough to deliver a lethal dose every four minutes to those who tried to fight the flames.

Some nuclear strategists see the nuclear winter effect as a strong argument for building defenses against bombers, cruise missiles, and ballistic missiles. Defensive systems, such as those envisaged under the proposed Strategic Defense Initiative, would—to the extent they were successful—reduce the number of warheads exploding on American territory. If the Soviet Union had failed to winterize its arsenal, the Strategic Defense Initiative would offer some compensation in preventing a Soviet attack from inducing nuclear winter.

Nuclear Winter and Arms Control

Others believe that the most important implication of nuclear winter is that the superpowers should urgently negotiate to bring their combined stockpile of nuclear weapons down to below the threshold numbers that could trigger climatic exchange. Carl Sagan, one of the five coauthors of the article that first described nuclear winter, suggests that the threshold lies at between 500 and 2,000 warheads. "To me," Sagan writes, "it seems clear that the species is in grave danger at least until the world arsenals are reduced below the threshold for climatic catastrophe. . . . If world arsenals were well below this rough threshold, no concatenation of computer malfunction, carelessness, unauthorized acts, communications failure, miscalculation and madness in high office could unleash nuclear winter."[8]

Nuclear strategists tend to oppose this interpretation. A principal objection is that a small arsenal would be destabilizing because an aggressor might be tempted to destroy it in a first strike. Leon Sloss, who directed the review of targeting policy that led to President Carter's PD-59, considers such an approach to be "impractical"—first, because no one knows where the threshold lies and, second, because two decades of strenuous negotiations with the Soviet Union have failed to secure major reductions of strategic arms.[9]

Even if a threshold level of nuclear stockpiles were desirable, negotiating a verifiable treaty to enforce it would require an unprecedented degree of openness from both parties, particularly the Soviet Union. Arms talks have hitherto dealt only in relatively crude measures of nuclear force, such as numbers and kinds of missiles and missile throw weight. These are quantities that can be verified by satellites and other independent means. But for the superpowers to negotiate arms reductions to minimize nuclear winter, notes a study by the Palomar Corporation of Washington, D.C., "the two sides might have to negotiate targeting restrictions, controls on fusing options and warhead-yield limitations—unlikely subjects for bilateral discussions much less negotiations. Targeting and fusing options are inherently non-verifiable."[10]

Preventing Nuclear War

There is already abundant incentive to avoid nuclear war. Yet the new understanding of the physical effects of a nuclear exchange, including nuclear winter, lends still further urgency to reducing the likelihood of all possible paths to nuclear war, particularly the risk of an unintended escalation in crisis to a preemptive first strike.

Probably the most important element in preventing a nuclear war is to maintain a credible nuclear deterrent. That requires repairing weaknesses that might tempt an opponent, in crisis, to gamble on the success of a preemptive first strike. The principal defects in America's nuclear deterrent lie in the softness of its nuclear command and control systems and in the vulnerability of its land-based missiles.

For two decades American governments have sought to reduce the risk of nuclear war through arms control agreements with the Soviet Union. Arms control has succeeded in many important aspects, notably in providing for the agreed inviolability of reconnaissance satellites and for a framework in which the superpowers can at least discuss the structure of their respective arsenals. Without this amount of insight into the adversary's defenses and attitudes, each side would necessarily assume and prepare for the worst outcome.

Many look to arms control as a means of reducing nuclear weapons. By this criterion it has failed; the size of both sides' strategic nuclear forces has increased enormously under the SALT I and SALT II treaties. On the other hand, the Anti-Ballistic Missile Treaty of 1972 has precluded a race to deploy defenses against ballistic missiles, as well as an interactive competition between nuclear offense and defense.

The popular expectation of reductions, however, misses the point. Reductions in themselves are not necessarily good; cutting back the size of nuclear arsenals could make a first strike seem more likely to succeed, or force each side back to a policy of destroying cities rather than military targets.

The purpose of arms control should be to structure the nuclear forces of each side so as to minimize the chances of war. It is by this criterion that arms control has been such a disappointment. Under SALT II, the Soviet Union has built up a massive force of land-based missiles carrying multiple nuclear warheads. This force, at least in theory, is enough to destroy all American land-based missiles and probably to devastate the American command and control system. Yet the Soviet missiles are themselves vulnerable targets, since their protective silos are susceptible to nuclear attack. Because of that combination of lethality and vulnerability, Soviet commanders know the missiles must be used early in a nuclear exchange or face destruction. In times of crisis, as noted in chapter 2, rapid interaction between one side's measures and the other's responses might quickly escalate to the brink of a nuclear exchange, inducing fierce pressures to strike first. Pressure will be particularly intense on the side with the more vulnerable forces. Multiwarhead, land-based missiles are therefore seen as weapons that destabilize the nuclear equilibrium.

The major failure of arms control is that the Soviet Union has come to rely preponderantly on a force of destabilizing weapons. The promising design of the SALT process was first to set caps on various categories of strategic weapons and then to lower the caps. Because the United States had chosen to place more of its strategic missiles aboard invulnerable submarines, the Soviet Union was allowed a larger force of land-based missiles. But as the Soviets increased the accuracy of their warheads, they turned this numerical advantage into the ability to destroy American land-based missiles in their silos, without facing the same threat themselves. The Soviet Union will not readily give up this advantage. Even if it were to agree to a ratio of Soviet to American land-based missiles that eliminated this threat, its remaining missiles would still be destabilizing weapons. The SALT process thus offers little imminent prospect of achieving its principal purpose, a stabler structure of nuclear arsenals.

That is why the Strategic Defense Initiative (SDI) proposed by President Reagan is in some ways more promising than he has so far made it appear. The reason is as follows. Defenses against ballistic missiles are viewed by some analysts as destabilizing. They can serve not only to defend against a first strike but also—rather more effectively—to shield the perpetrator of a first strike against retaliation. Defenses also induce the other side to increase its offenses in order to ensure penetration. It was these arguments, at least on the American side, that prompted the signing of the ABM Treaty. Mr. Reagan's resurrection of the idea of strategic defenses in 1983 seemed to defy this logic for no clear purpose. His promise of a system that would defend the whole country against ballistic missiles was judged impossible by most experts. Further research has if anything amplified the apparent technical difficulties of nationwide defense. Initial public reaction to the Strategic Defense Initiative has been distinctly skeptical.

The program was greeted with rather more respect in the Soviet Union. Perhaps like many American analysts who support the Strategic Defense Initiative, the Soviets see in it a quite different purpose, that of defending missile silos and command posts against ballistic missiles. This is a far easier task than affording absolute protection to soft targets like cities, and indeed a defense program probably could provide credible limited coverage of military assets. Whether or not it was Mr. Reagan's intention, SDI appears to have afforded the United States considerable leverage in negotiations with the Soviet Union. Mikhail Gorbachev's paramount need is to revive his lagging economy, not to shift scarce resources and engineers into a massive competition in missile defenses. Apart from the MX missile, which Congress has refused to build in sufficiently threatening numbers, the Strategic Defense Initiative is perhaps the only implement that could have shifted the Soviet Union from its liking for the status quo of the SALT regime.

Yet even granting the crude leverage of the Strategic Defense Initiative, many experts still doubt its desirability. The Soviets can be pushed only so far from what they regard as their national interest. Instead of offering significant concessions, their response may be to open a costly race in both offensive and defensive systems that will leave neither side safer than before.

To this doubtful picture Reagan in 1986 added a new and startling ingredient. In a letter to Gorbachev and again at the Reykjavík summit, he proposed that both sides eliminate all their strategic ballistic missiles. This concept, also a radical departure from conventional strategic thinking, put the Strategic

Defense Initiative in an interesting new context. Together, the two proposals hold out the distant possibility, at least in theory, of a stabler structure of nuclear deterrence.

In Reagan's new world, each side would maintain nuclear weapons, but the means of delivery would be bombers and air-breathing cruise missiles (which in essence are unmanned bombers). Each would construct air defenses to shoot down bombers and cruise missiles. Even though ballistic missiles would be abolished, each superpower would be free to construct SDI defenses against them in case of cheating by the other side. SDI defenses would in fact be a critical feature of the Reagan world because, with the official elimination of ballistic missile forces, concealment of even a few weapons would confer a critical advantage. Probably neither side would agree to abandon its missiles until some form of defense system were in place as insurance against cheating.

What advantages might such a strategic structure offer? Unlike ballistic missiles, with a flight time of about 25 minutes, strategic bombers and cruise missiles take some six hours to reach their targets and even then can perhaps be met with credible defenses. This interval should allow far more time for decision making. Whereas land-based missiles may need to be fired promptly in an exchange to escape destruction, response against an attack by bombers and cruise missiles could be delayed much longer. In the case of an escalation of nuclear alerts during a crisis, the tremendous pressure on leaders to launch a preemptive strike would be considerably lessened.

For the United States, such a world would mean riddance of the greatest threat to American security and to a stable nuclear balance—the Soviet Union's destabilizing force of multiwarhead, land-based missiles. For the Soviet Union, the arrangement would mean freedom from fear of the almost certain American advantage in ballistic missile defense since, without ballistic missiles, such defenses would shed their ambiguous nature and become purely defensive.

Far more analysis is needed to know if the Reagan vision of nuclear deterrence without ballistic missiles would indeed lead out of the dangerous impasse of SALT and toward a stabler world. The temptation to cheating would be considerably greater than at present and its consequences more profound. The receding danger of nuclear war could in fact make such war more likely, by encouraging brinkmanship or by failing to deter a precipitating conventional war between the superpowers. Nonetheless, the proposal is worth exploring, and could prove a promising long-term goal. Attaining it is another matter.

Arms control agreements require assent between the superpowers. But there are many measures to enhance strategic stability that can be undertaken by one side acting alone. Installation by the United States of Permissive Action Links on its nuclear weapons has greatly reduced the risk of nuclear war by accidental or unauthorized launch. Conversion of the land-based missile force from silo basing to mobile launchers would make it less vulnerable and therefore more stabilizing. The mobile Midgetman missile, designed to carry one or more warheads, will be a significant step in this direction. As previously noted, protecting command and control systems against nuclear attack, particularly by hardening them against the effects of the electromagnetic pulse, would strengthen the United States at its weakest point and one that most invites attack. The Reagan Administration has made a special effort in this vital but unglamorous task.

The structure of nuclear deterrence has been stable for more than 40 years. But that in no way guarantees another 40 years of stability. Nuclear arsenals have changed greatly during this period. The United States enjoyed an overwhelming superiority in nuclear arms until the mid-1970s. The Soviet Union has now attained overall parity, and an advantage in what strategists call prompt, hard-target kill capability—meaning missiles that can knock out other missiles in their silos. Just as a seesaw is at its most precarious when evenly balanced, so the present state of nuclear parity is less stable than the former state of American superiority. Regaining American superiority is not necessarily desirable. Even if it were, popular support for such a course would be unlikely. Therefore the other routes to nuclear stability must be explored all the more urgently. The structure of nuclear deterrence still looks sound. But until it is tested in crisis, no one can be sure it will not be liable to catastrophic failure.

The Failure of Nuclear Deterrence

The blocking of all conceivable paths to nuclear war is a vital strategy for the immediate future. In the longer term, it is the policy of nuclear deterrence that must be replaced.

Present doctrine commits the United States, in the name of deterrence, to prepare for a protracted nuclear war. No one knows how or whether such a war could be fought. Many believe that once the first nuclear weapons are exploded, nothing will stop an escalation up to a full exchange.

No one knows if the Soviet Union, the supposed partner in the doctrine's concept of negotiated nuclear war, has any intention of playing its assigned role. Publicly at least, the Soviet Union ridicules the strategists' notions of nuclear war fighting. Marshal N. V. Ogarkov wrote in 1984, "The calculation of the strategists across the ocean, based on the possibility of waging a so-called 'limited' nuclear war, now has no foundation whatever. It is utopian: Any so-called limited use of nuclear forces will inevitably lead to the immediate use of the whole of the sides' nuclear arsenals. This is the terrible logic of war."[11]

Despite the years of analysis that nuclear strategists have spent constructing the theory of flexible response, concludes Fred Kaplan, the doctrine is merely a "compelling illusion." "Even many of those who recognized its pretense and inadequacy willingly fell under its spell. They continued to play the game because there was no other. They performed their calculations and spoke in their strange and esoteric tongues because to do otherwise would be to recognize, all too clearly and constantly, the ghastliness of their contemplations. They contrived their options because without them the bomb would appear too starkly as the thing that they had tried to prevent it from being but that it ultimately would become if it ever were used—a device of sheer mayhem, a weapon whose cataclysmic powers no one really had the faintest idea of how to control. The nuclear strategists had come to impose order—but in the end, chaos still prevailed."[12]

With each struggle to find new answers, the first question of the nuclear age becomes ever more intractable. What if deterrence fails? Fighting a war to negotiate a cease-fire short of absolute destruction is better than nothing but is slender insurance against catastrophe. Nuclear deterrence has succeeded so far, but the full price of failure has never been clearly acknowledged, because governments did not seek to learn it. With the discovery of the possibility of nuclear winter and other consequences, the likely result of failure turns out to be still worse than imagined.

If the consequences of nuclear war make that risk intolerable, then alternatives must be sought to the policy of nuclear deterrence. Abandonment of nuclear arms without other change would be no solution, merely a recipe for conventional war, sooner or later, between the superpowers. The necessary change must come in the state of tension that gives each superpower cause to fear the other.

Such peaceful evolution is unlikely to happen overnight. Nuclear deterrence must last until it does. With the new knowledge of the consequences of nuclear weapons, the United States and the Soviet Union must reconsider the calculus of terror and strive for a form of coexistence that does not require the present world's destruction as its guarantee.

Notes

Chapter 1
Under the Shadow

1. Richard K. Betts, *Surprise Attack: Lessons for Defense Planning* (Washington, D.C.: Brookings Institution, 1982), 248.
2. John D. Steinbruner, "Managerial Demands of Modern Weapons Systems," in *The Medical Implications of Nuclear War* (Washington, D.C.: National Academy Press, 1986).
3. Alexander L. George, "The Impact of Crisis-Induced Stress on Decision-making," in *Medical Implications of Nuclear War.*
4. Ibid.

Chapter 2
The Fragilities of Command and Control

1. John M. Collins, *US-Soviet Military Balance, 1980–1985* (Washington, D.C.: Congressional Research Service, 1985), 313.
2. Ibid., 305, 308; Bruce G. Blair, *Strategic Command and Control* (Washington, D.C.: Brookings Institution, 1985), 310.
3. The description of the nuclear command and control system is drawn from Blair, *Strategic Command and Control,* and from Paul Bracken, *The Command and Control of Nuclear Forces* (New Haven: Yale University Press, 1983).
4. Paul Bracken, "Accidental Nuclear War," in *Hawks, Doves, and Owls,* ed. Graham T. Allison et al. (New York: Norton, 1985), 40.
5. Donald R. Cotter, "Peacetime Operations," in *Managing Nuclear Operations* (Washington, D.C.: Brookings Institution, 1987).
6. Ibid.

7. John D. Steinbruner, "Managerial Demands of Modern Weapons Systems," in *Medical Implications of Nuclear War.*

8. Bracken, *Command and Control of Nuclear Forces,* 53.

9. Stephen M. Meyer, "Soviet Perspectives on the Paths to Nuclear War," in *Hawks, Doves, and Owls,* 188–89.

10. Blair, *Strategic Command and Control,* 182.

11. Ibid., 283, 294.

12. John D. Steinbruner, "Launch under Attack," *Scientific American,* January 1984, 37–47.

13. Blair, *Strategic Command and Control,* 239.

14. John D. Steinbruner, "An Assessment of Nuclear Crises," in *The Dangers of Nuclear War,* ed. Franklyn Griffiths and John C. Polyani (Toronto: University of Toronto Press, 1979), 38.

15. Bracken, *Command and Control of Nuclear Forces,* 48.

CHAPTER 3
Flash, Blast, and Fire

1. Samuel Glasstone and Philip J. Dolan, *The Effects of Nuclear Weapons,* 3d ed. (Washington, D.C.: Department of Defense, 1977), 28. Parameters for the effects of nuclear weapons are taken from this standard source or from Theodore A. Postol, "Possible Fatalities from Superfires following Nuclear Attacks in or near Urban Areas," in *The Medical Implications of Nuclear War* (Washington, D.C.: National Academy Press, 1986).

2. Bruce G. Blair, *Strategic Command and Control* (Washington, D.C.: Brookings Institution, 1985), 310.

3. Committee for the Compilation of Materials on Damage Caused by the Atomic Bombs in Hiroshima and Nagasaki, *Hiroshima and Nagasaki,* trans. Eisei Ishikawa and David L. Swain (New York: Basic Books, 1981). Details of the Hiroshima and Nagasaki bombings are drawn from this source and from Glasstone and Dolan, *Effects of Nuclear Weapons,* unless otherwise mentioned.

4. Pacific War Research Society, *The Day Man Lost* (Tokyo: Kodansha International, 1981), 238–42.

5. Ibid., 247–49.

6. Ashley W. Oughterson and Shields Warren, *Medical Effects of the Atomic Bomb in Japan* (New York: McGraw-Hill, 1956), 86.

7. Committee for the Compilation, *Hiroshima and Nagasaki,* 113–14.

8. Oughterson and Warren, *Medical Effects,* 86.

9. Fred Kaplan, *The Wizards of Armageddon* (New York: Simon & Schuster, 1983), 36.

10. Ronald H. Spector, *Eagle against the Sun* (New York: Macmillan, 1984), 505.

11. Stephen E. Ambrose, *Eisenhower,* vol. 1 (New York: Simon & Schuster, 1983), 426.

12. Spector, *Eagle against the Sun,* 555.

13. H. L. Brode and R. D. Small, "A Review of the Physics of Large Urban Fires," in *Medical Implications of Nuclear War.*

14. John W. Birks and Sherry L. Stephens, "Possible Toxic Environments following a Nuclear War," in *Medical Implications of Nuclear War.*

15. Postol, "Possible Fatalities."

CHAPTER 4

Fallout

1. Samuel Glasstone and Philip J. Dolan, *The Effects of Nuclear Weapons,* 3d ed. (Washington, D.C.: Department of Defense, 1977), 42.

2. Ibid., 436–39, 602–3.

3. Committee for the Compilation of Materials on Damage Caused by the Atomic Bombs in Hiroshima and Nagasaki, *Hiroshima and Nagasaki,* trans. Eisei Ishikawa and David L. Swain (New York: Basic Books, 1981), 575.

4. Charles S. Shapiro et al., "Radioactive Fallout," in *The Medical Implications of Nuclear War* (Washington, D.C.: National Academy Press, 1986).

5. Ibid.

6. L. Devell et al., "Initial Observations of Fallout from the Reactor Accident at Chernobyl," *Nature* 321 (1986): 192–93.

7. Tim Beardsley, "US Analysis Incomplete," *Nature* 321 (1986): 187.

8. William J. Broad, "Experts Voice Concern on East Europe Cancers," *New York Times,* 16 May 1986, A6.

CHAPTER 5

The Medical Effects of Nuclear War

1. Samuel Glasstone and Philip J. Dolan, *The Effects of Nuclear Weapons,* 3d ed. (Washington, D.C.: Department of Defense, 1977), 549.

2. Ibid.

3. Ibid., 563.

4. Ibid., 569.

5. Ibid., 571.

6. Committee for the Compilation of Materials on Damage Caused by the Atomic Bombs in Hiroshima and Nagasaki, *Hiroshima and Nagasaki,* trans. Eisei Ishikawa and David L. Swain (New York: Basic Books, 1981), 130–31, 148.

7. Glasstone and Dolan, *Effects of Nuclear Weapons,* 579.

8. Ibid., 580–81; J. E. Coggle and Patricia J. Lindop, "Medical Consequences of Radiation following a Global Nuclear War," *Ambio* 11 (1982): 106–13.

9. Joseph Rotblat, "Acute Radiation Mortality in a Nuclear War," in *The Medical Implications of Nuclear War* (Washington, D.C.: National Academy Press, 1986).

10. Ashley W. Oughterson and Shields Warren, *Medical Effects of the Atomic Bomb in Japan* (New York: McGraw-Hill, 1956), 81.

11. Committee for the Compilation, *Hiroshima and Nagasaki*, 379.

12. Ibid., 382.

13. Herbert L. Abrams, "Medical Supply and Demand in the Post–Nuclear War World," in *Medical Implications of Nuclear War.*

14. Committee for the Compilation, *Hiroshima and Nagasaki*, 532.

15. Oughterson and Warren, *Medical Effects*, 82.

16. Glasstone and Dolan, *Effects of Nuclear Weapons*, 391.

17. James Thompson, "Psychological Consequences of Disaster: Analogies for the Nuclear Case," in *Medical Implications of Nuclear War.*

18. Michihiko Hachiya, *Hiroshima Diary* (Chapel Hill: University of North Carolina Press, 1955), 54–55.

19. Robert Jay Lifton and Kai Erikson, "Survivors of Nuclear War: Psychological and Communal Breakdown," in *Last Aid: The Medical Dimensions of Nuclear War*, ed. Eric Chivian et al. (San Francisco: W. H. Freeman, 1982), 292.

20. Klaus G. Wetzel, "Effects on Global Supplies of Fresh Water," *Ambio* 11 (1982): 126–31.

21. H. Kato and I. Shigematsu, "Late Effects of A-Bomb Radiation: Hiroshima and Nagasaki," in *Effects of Nuclear War on Health and Health Services* (Geneva: World Health Organization, 1984), 128.

22. Ibid., 121.

23. Glasstone and Dolan, *Effects of Nuclear Weapons*, 593. The estimate is in fact ten extra cases per rem of exposure. A rem is equivalent to a rad for many types of radiation, including gamma rays and neutrons at certain energies.

24. C. E. Land and Per Oftedal, "Cancer Induction as a Result of Nuclear War," in *Effects of Nuclear War on Health*, 147–61.

25. Glasstone and Dolan, *Effects of Nuclear Weapons*, 613. The actual estimate is 50 *rems* (see n. 23).

26. Per Oftedal, "Genetic Damage following Nuclear War," in *Effects of Nuclear War on Health*, 163–72.

27. William J. Shull, Masanori Otake, and James V. Neel, "Genetic Effects of the Atomic Bombs: A Reappraisal," *Science* 213 (1981): 1220–27.

CHAPTER 6

Nuclear War and Climate

1. *Long-term Worldwide Effects of Multiple Nuclear-Weapons Detonations* (Washington, D.C.: National Academy of Sciences, 1975).

2. Paul J. Crutzen and John W. Birks, "The Atmosphere after a Nuclear War: Twilight at Noon," *Ambio* 11 (1982): 114–25.

3. R. P. Turco et al., "Nuclear Winter: Global Consequences of Multiple Nuclear Explosions," *Science* 222 (1983): 1283–92.

4. Edward Teller, "Widespread After-effects of Nuclear War," *Nature* 310 (1984): 621–24.

5. *The Effects on the Atmosphere of a Major Nuclear Exchange* (Washington, D.C.: National Academy of Sciences, 1985), 1.

6. Albert Wohlstetter, "Between an Unfree World and None," *Foreign Affairs* 63 (1985): 962–94.

7. George F. Carrier, "Nuclear Winter: An Overview of Atmospheric Changes," *Issues in Science and Technology*, Winter 1985, 114–17.

8. Robert C. Malone et al., "Nuclear Winter: Three-dimensional Simulations including Interactive Transport, Scavenging and Solar Heating of Smoke" (submitted to the *Journal of Geophysical Research*).

9. Ibid.

10. Starley L. Thompson and Stephen H. Schneider, "Nuclear Winter Reapraised," *Foreign Affairs* 64 (1986): 981–1005.

11. Scientific Committee on Problems of the Environment, *Environmental Consequences of Nuclear War*, vol. 1, *Physical and Atmospheric Effects* (New York: John Wiley, 1985).

CHAPTER 7
The Havoc Factor and the Ozone Shield

1. Samuel Glasstone and Philip J. Dolan, *The Effects of Nuclear Weapons*, 3d ed. (Washington, D.C.: Department of Defense, 1977), 519.

2. *Evaluation of Methodologies for Estimating Vulnerability to Electromagnetic Pulse Effects* (Washington, D.C.: National Academy of Sciences, 1984).

3. William J. Broad, "The Chaos Factor," *Science 83*, January/February 1983, 41–49.

4. Scientific Committee on the Problems of the Environment, *Environmental Consequences of Nuclear War*, vol. 1, *Physical and Atmospheric Effects* (New York: John Wiley, 1985), 18.

5. *Evaluation of Methodologies.*

6. Broad, "Chaos Factor."

7. Bruce G. Blair, *Strategic Command and Control* (Washington, D.C.: Brookings Institution, 1985), appendix D.

8. Lydia Dotto and Harold Schiff, *The Ozone War* (New York: Doubleday, 1978).

9. *The Effects on the Atmosphere of a Major Nuclear Exchange* (Washington, D.C.: National Academy of Sciences, 1985).

10. Ibid., 108.

11. *Long-term Worldwide Effects of Multiple Nuclear-Weapons Detonations* (Washington, D.C.: National Academy of Sciences, 1975).

12. *Effects on the Atmosphere.*

13. John W. Birks and Sherry L. Stephens, "Possible Toxic Environments following a Nuclear War," in *The Medical Implications of Nuclear War* (Washington, D.C.: National Academy Press, 1986).

14. Scientific Committee, *Environmental Consequences of Nuclear War*, 1:218.

CHAPTER 8
Agriculture and Environment after War

1. *Long-term Worldwide Effects of Multiple Nuclear-Weapons Detonations* (Washington, D.C.: National Academy of Sciences, 1985), 96.

2. Ibid., i–vi.

3. Richard B. Stothers, "The Great Tambora Eruption and Its Aftermath," *Science* 224 (1984): 1191–98.

4. *Long-term Worldwide Effects*, 94.

5. Mark A. Harwell and Christine C. Harwell, "Nuclear Famine: The Indirect Effects of Nuclear War," in *The Medical Implications of Nuclear War* (Washington, D.C.: National Academy Press, 1986).

6. *Long-term Worldwide Effects*.

7. Scientific Committee on the Problems of the Environment, *Environmental Consequences of Nuclear War*, vol. 1, *Physical and Atmospheric Effects* (New York: John Wiley, 1985), 201.

8. Scientific Committee on the Problems of the Environment, *Environmental Consequences of Nuclear War*, vol. 2, *Ecological and Agricultural Effects* (New York: John Wiley, 1985), 318–19.

9. Alexander Leaf, "Food and Nutrition in the Aftermath of a Nuclear War," in *Medical Implications of Nuclear War*.

10. Mark A. Harwell, *Nuclear Winter* (New York: Springer Verlag, 1985), 130.

11. Scientific Committee, *Environmental Consequences of Nuclear War*, 2:483.

12. The following section is based on the discussion in chapters 1–3 of the assessment of the biological effects of nuclear war compiled by the Scientific Committee on the Problems of the Environment, a body supported by the International Council of Scientific Unions.

CHAPTER 9
Casualties and Survivors

1. Office of Technology Assessment, *The Effects of Nuclear War* (Washington, D.C.: Government Printing Office, 1979).

2. William Daugherty, Barbara Levi, and Frank von Hippel, "The Consequences of 'Limited' Nuclear Attacks on the US," in *The Medical Implications of Nuclear War* (Washington, D.C.: National Academy Press, 1986).

3. Alexander Leaf, "Food and Nutrition in the Aftermath of a Nuclear War," in *Medical Implications of Nuclear War*.

4. Yves Laulan, "Economic Consequences: Back to the Dark Ages," *Ambio* 11 (1982): 149–52.

5. Hal Cochrane and Dennis Mileti, "The Consequences of Nuclear War: An Economic and Social Perspective," in *Medical Implications of Nuclear War.*

CHAPTER 10
Rethinking Nuclear War

1. Leon Sloss and Marc D. Millot, "U.S. Nuclear Strategy in Evolution," *Strategic Review,* Winter 1984, 19–28.

2. Caspar W. Weinberger, *Report of the Secretary of Defense Caspar W. Weinberger to the Congress* (Washington, D.C.: Government Printing Office, 1984), 29–30.

3. Robert Scheer, *With Enough Shovels* (New York: Random House, 1982), 3, 21.

4. Michael M. May, "Nuclear Winter: Strategic Significance," *Issues in Science and Technology,* Winter 1985, 118–20.

5. *Nuclear Winter and Its Implications: Hearings before the Committee on Armed Services, U.S. Senate, October 2 and 3, 1985* (Washington, D.C.: Government Printing Office, 1985).

6. Theodore A. Postol, "Strategic Confusion—with or without Nuclear Winter," *Bulletin of Atomic Scientists,* February 1985, 14–17.

7. Francis P. Hoeber and Robert K. Squire, "The 'Nuclear Winter' Hypothesis: Some Policy Implications," *Strategic Review,* Summer 1985, 39–46.

8. Carl Sagan, "Nuclear War and Climatic Catastrophe: Some Policy Implications," *Foreign Affairs* 62 (1983–84): 257–92.

9. Leon Sloss, *Nuclear Winter and Its Implications: Hearings before the Committee on Armed Services, U.S. Senate, October 2 and 3, 1985* (Washington, D.C.: Government Printing Office, 1985).

10. *Implications of the "Nuclear Winter" Thesis: Report Prepared for the Defense Nuclear Agency* (Washington, D.C.: Palomar Corp., 1985).

11. Quoted in Leon Goure, " 'Nuclear Winter' in Soviet Mirrors," *Strategic Review,* Summer 1985, 22–38.

12. Fred Kaplan, *Wizards of Armageddon,* (New York: Simon & Schuster, 1983), 390.

Index

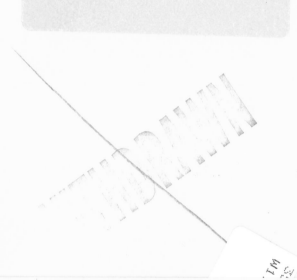